AF079423

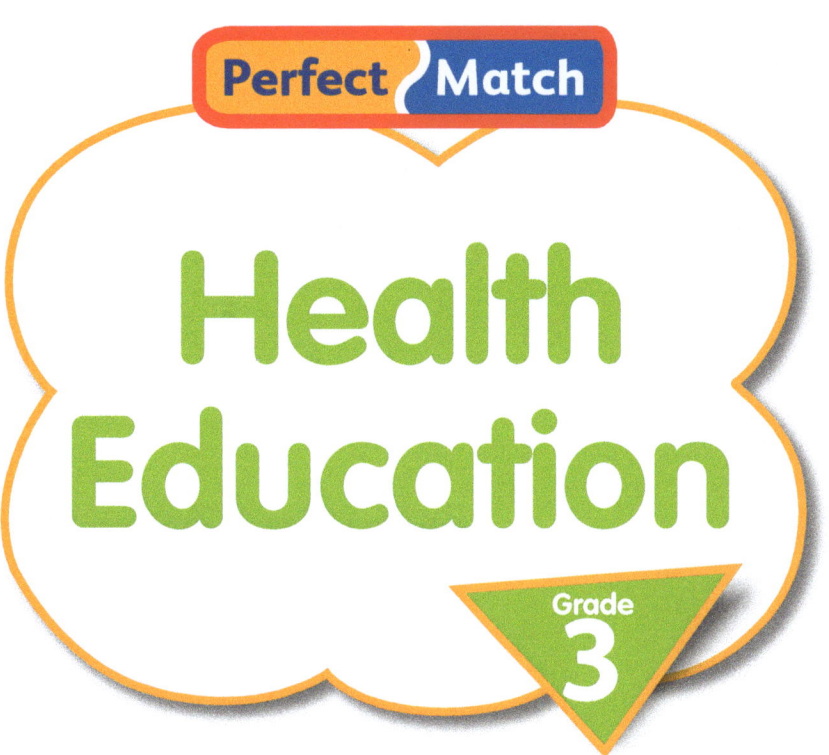

Dr Michael Chia

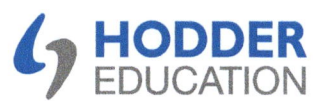

Contents

Physical Health

Lesson	Title	Page
1	Good Eating Habits	3
2	My Healthy Plate	5
3	Food Detective	9
4	Am I Eating Right?	11
5	Stay Active	15
6	A Dip In The Pool	17
7	Should Lam Accept The Offer?	19
8	Look At Our Posters	21
9	Give Your Eyes A Break	23
10	Something To Chew On	25

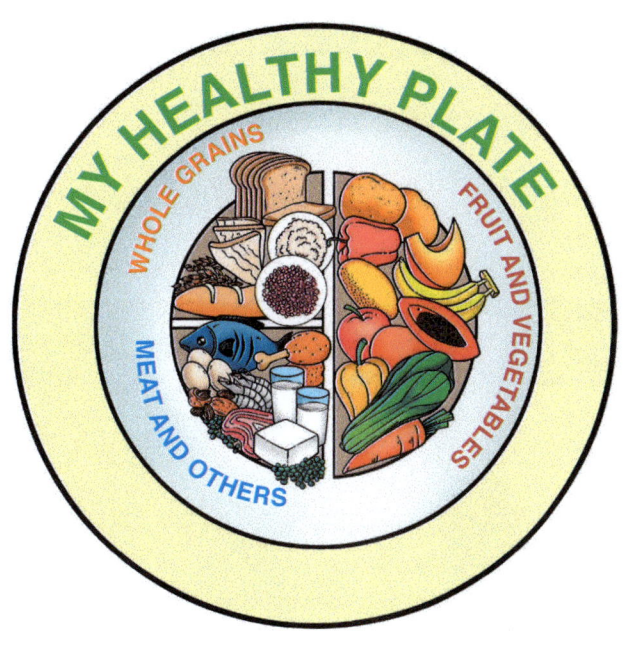

Environment And Your Health

Lesson	Title	Page
1	A Picnic	29
2	Trouble In The Kitchen	31
3	Kitchen Hygiene	33
4 & 5	No More Mosquitoes	35

Emotional And Psychological Health

Lesson	Title	Page
1	I Do Not Agree	43
2	Would You Get Angry?	45
3	What Started It?	47
4	Resolving Conflicts	49
5	No More Conflicts	51
6	I Do Not Feel Good	53
7	Same Or Different?	55
8	I Am Special	57
9	The Good, Bad And Ugly	59
10	My Special Shield	61
11	Building Relationships	63

Learning Log   65-70

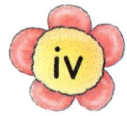

Introduction to the Pupil's Book

The **Perfect Match** Primary Health Education Pupil's Book is a full-colour textbook-cum-activity book. It contains lessons based on topics from the three dimensions in Health Education: Physical Health, Environment and Your Health, and Emotional and Psychological Health.

The book is organised by dimension and is presented in the order stated above. The pages in each dimension are colour-coded for easy reference.

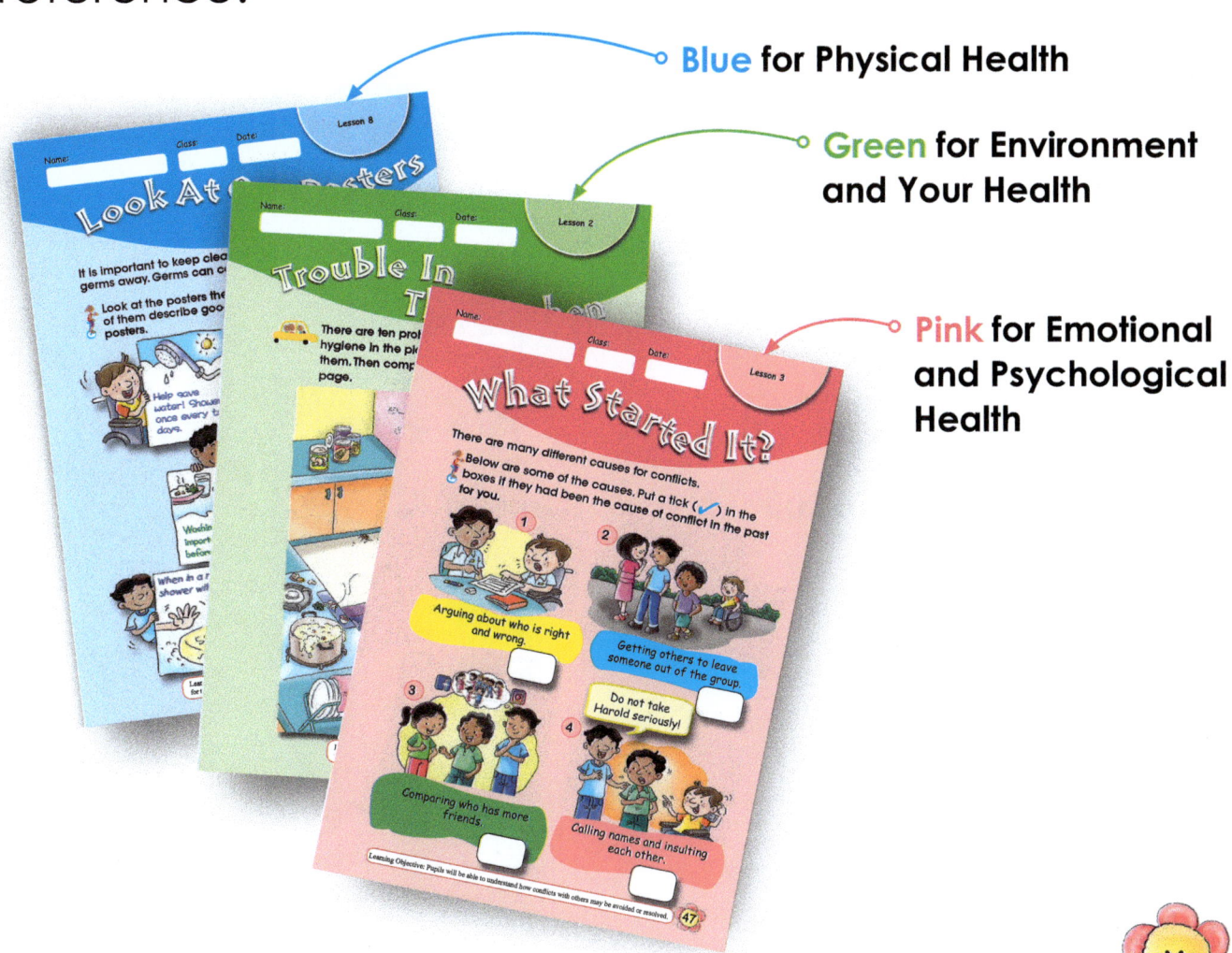

Blue for Physical Health

Green for Environment and Your Health

Pink for Emotional and Psychological Health

The Pupil's Book contains a variety of activities such as role plays, surveys, songs, matching exercises and craft work. In addition, there is a mix of activities requiring work in pairs, in groups or with the class.

Four icons indicate the nature of the activity to be conducted.

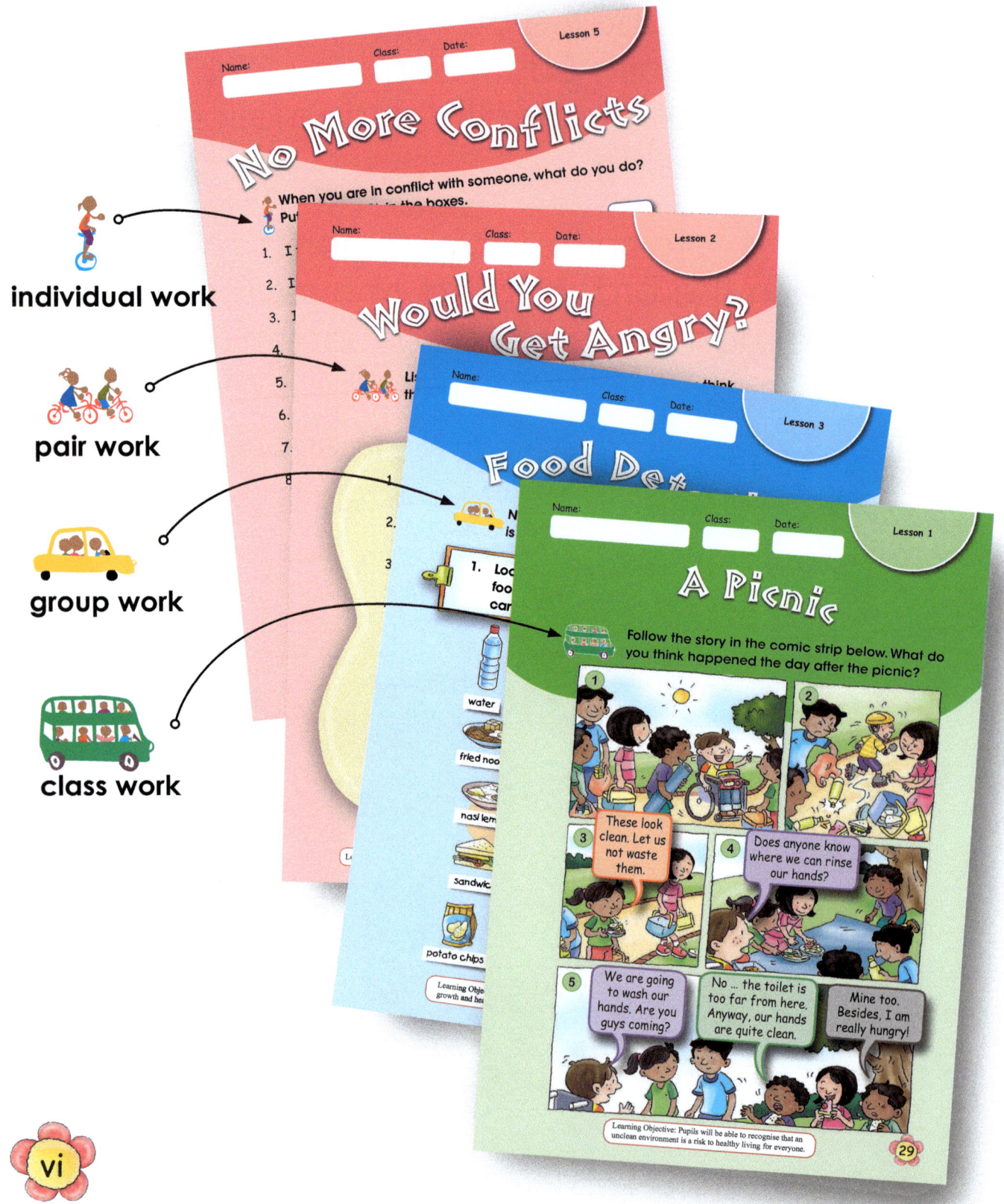

individual work

pair work

group work

class work

Difficult terms mentioned in the text are explained through a feature signalled by the dictionary icon.

The learning objective(s) for each lesson is/are listed for parents' and teachers' reference.

A dictionary icon signals the explanation of any difficult term(s) found on the page.

The learning objective(s) for each lesson is/are indicated at the opening page of each lesson.

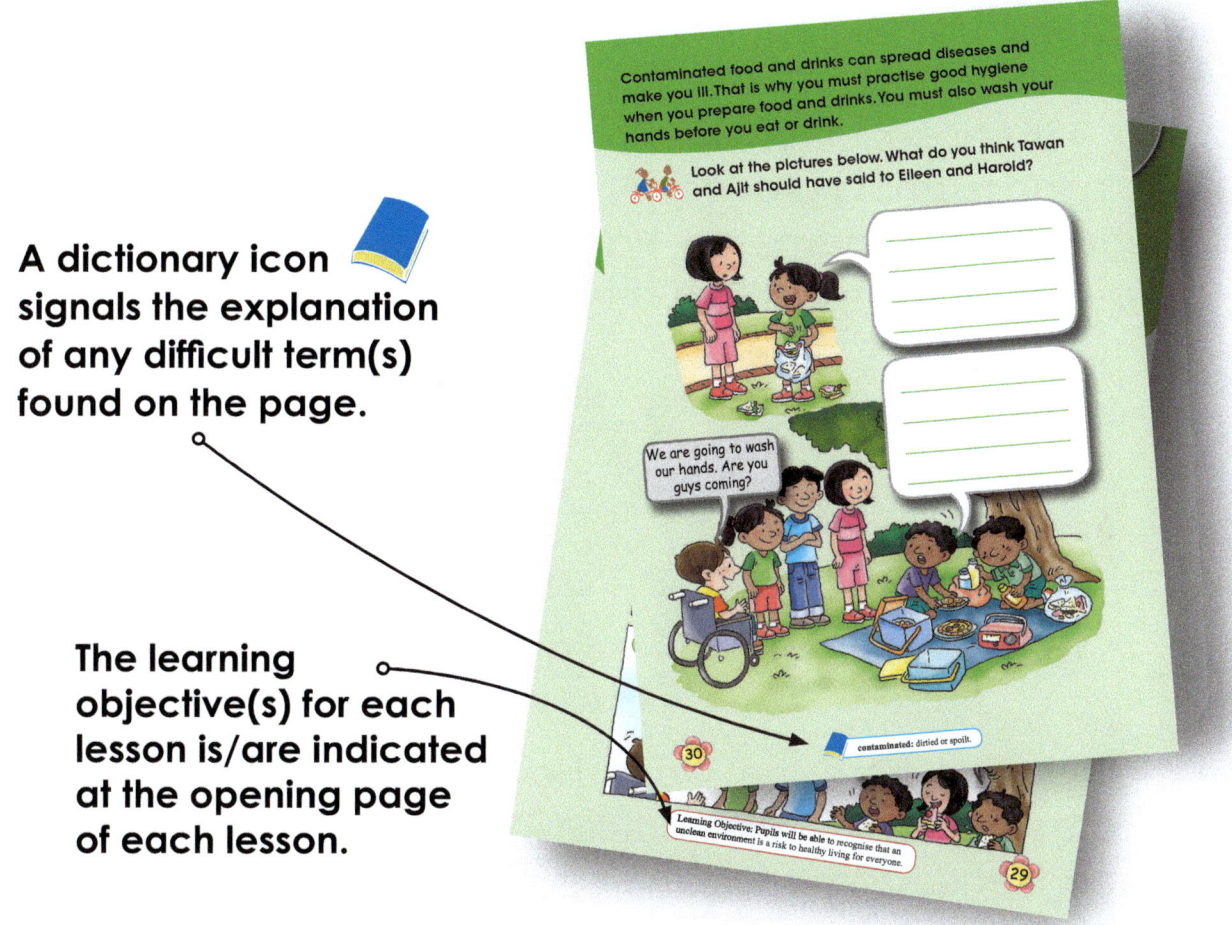

A Note on Short Forms: In the first three books, short-forms of verbs are avoided as early users of the language may not have knowledge of them. In Books 4, 5 and 6, these contractions are present throughout so that the language flows more naturally and pupils can become more acquainted with real English use.

A Learning Log has been added at the end of the book to give opportunity for reflective learning.

Introduction to the Superfriends

The materials in the Perfect Match **Perfect Match** Primary Health Education Pupil's Book revolve around six superfriends from some of the ASEAN countries. These six friends will accompany the pupils in the learning process as they move from Book 1 to 6. The first letters of their names — Haris, Eileen, Ajit, Lam, Tawan and Harold — form the word 'h-e-a-l-t-h'.

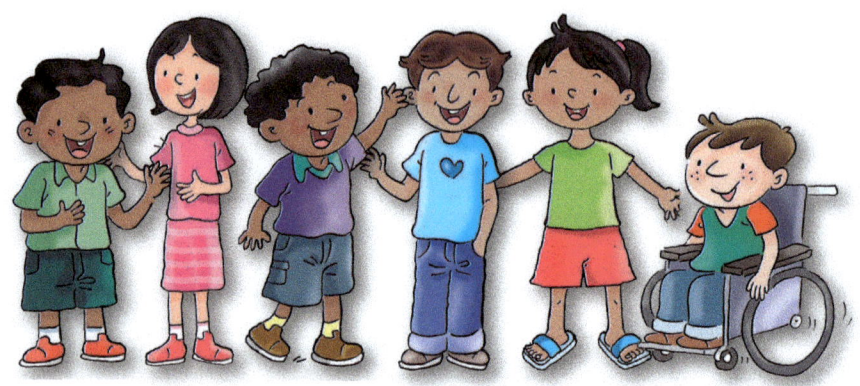

Taking the cue from the World Health Organization (WHO) to build 'a better and healthier future for people all over the world', the superfriends come together from different ASEAN countries to help young people like themselves develop healthy habits to ensure a better future. This health series aims to help pupils start early in health education, to keep themselves well physically, psychologically and emotionally. In addition, they will also learn to behave responsibly in order to enhance the environment in their home countries.

Hi, I am Haris.

Haris is a well-built Malaysian boy. He is the wise one among the superfriends. He is fun and peace-loving and tries his best to keep the people around him happy.

"Hi, I am Eileen."

Eileen is a tall slim Singaporean girl. She loves Maths and Science and knows a lot about computers. Eileen enjoys helping her friends with school work.

"Hi, I am Ajit."

Ajit is a Malaysian boy who loves reading and has a flair for languages. He speaks well and is always eager to listen to his friends when they have problems.

"Hi, I am Lam."

Lam is a Vietnamese boy who is active and full of ideas. He loves school and hopes to be a teacher when he grows up. He is good-natured and patient and is extremely well-liked.

Hi, I am Tawan.

Tawan is an athletic and sporty Thai girl who also loves art. She is the most physically active and well-rounded person in the group. She is smart and strong in character but also fun-loving and witty.

Hi, I am Harold.

Harold has a Canadian father and a biracial mother who is half Singaporean. He is musically talented and has great willpower. Despite his disability, he has never felt disadvantaged and he always encourages his friends to pursue their interests.

About The Author

Dr Michael Chia is Professor of Paediatric Exercise Science at the Physical Education & Sports Science Group in the National Institute of Education (NIE), Nanyang Technological University (NTU). He is an established author in the field of Health Education, Physical Education and Sports Science.

His health education publications include *Healthy, Well and Wise: Take PRIDE For A Life of Wellness*, *Invest in Better Health* and *Treks: All Aboard!*.

Physical Health

In this section, you will learn:

- some good eating habits;
- about My Healthy Plate;
- how good hygiene prevents illnesses and diseases;
- how to take care of your eyes; and
- about types of food that are good for your teeth and bones.

Name: Class: Date: Lesson 1

Good Eating Habits

Lam, Eileen, Harold, Ajit and their families are at an exhibition about good eating habits. Listen carefully as your teacher reads. Fill in the blanks.

Look, Grandpa, it says here that having regular meals keeps you healthy. It means we should have b _ _ _ _ _ _ _ _ _ _, l _ _ _ _ _ and d _ _ _ _ _ _ every day. It also says we are to eat a little of a wide variety of food.

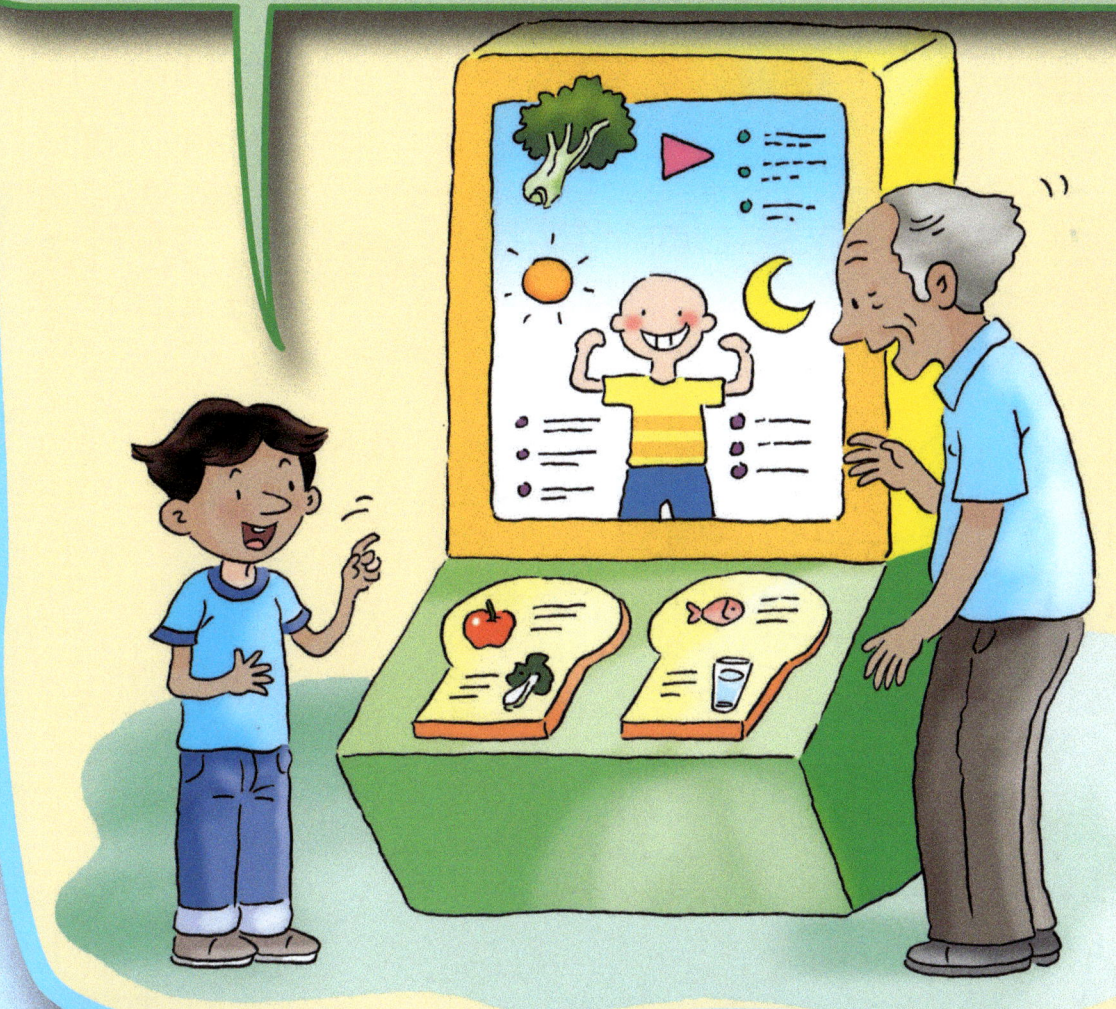

Learning Objective: Pupils will be able to make healthy food choices to obtain and maintain healthy growth.

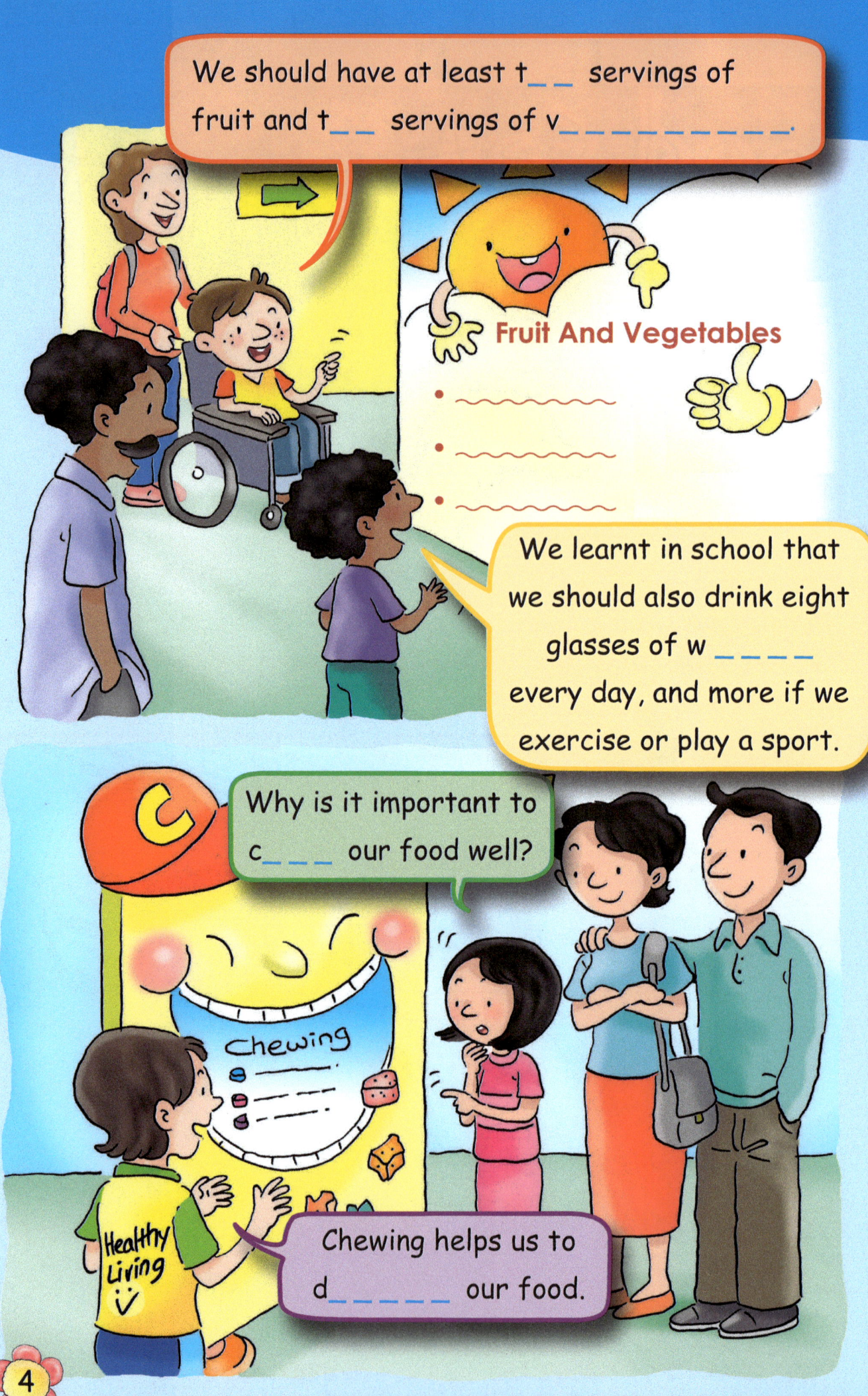

Name: Class: Date:

Lessons 2

My Healthy Plate

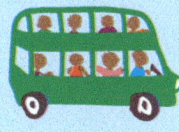 The picture shows My Healthy Plate—an easy guide to eating balanced and healthy meals. Can you name some of the food from the different food groups?

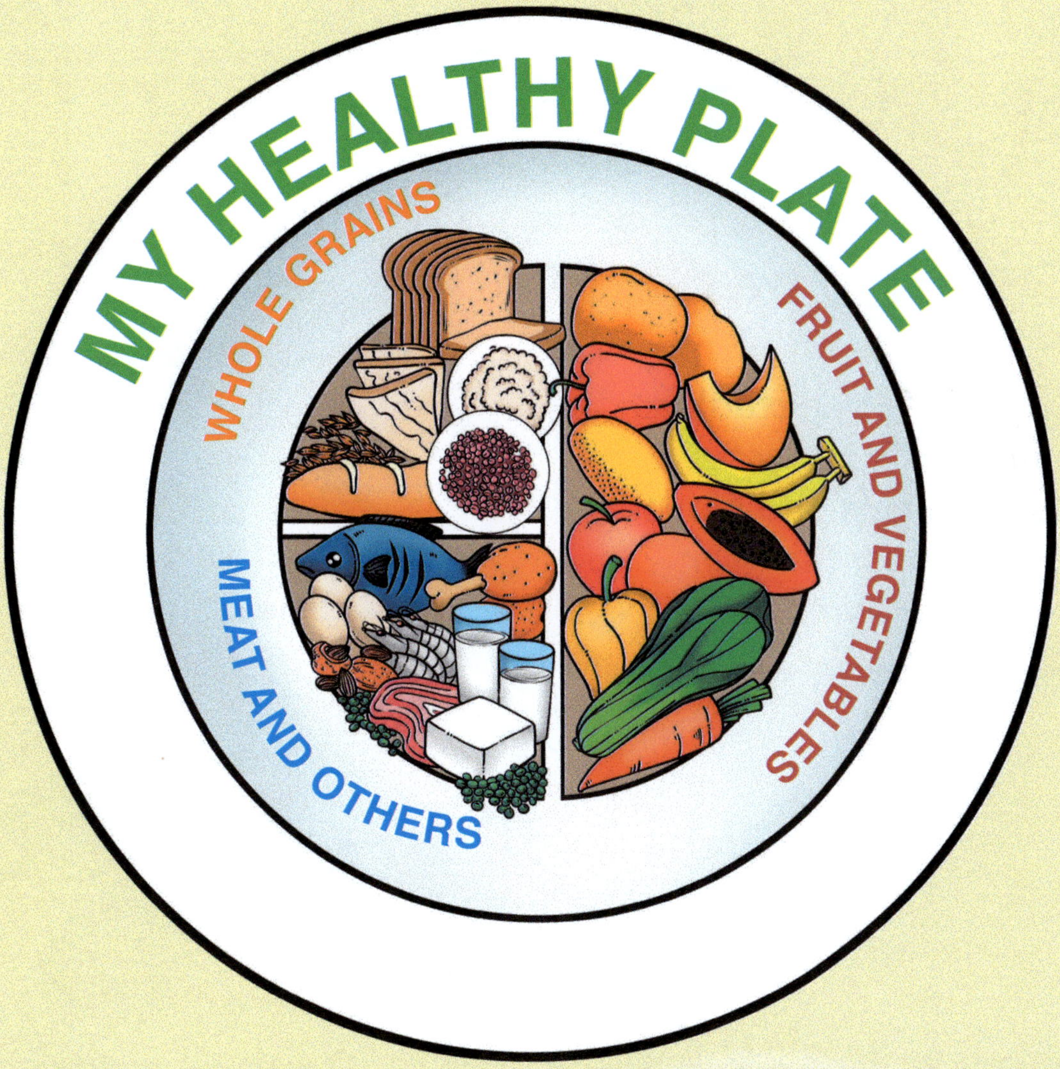

Learning Objectives: Pupils will be able to identify the different types of food for growth and health, and make healthy food choices to obtain and maintain healthy growth.

There are three food groups in My Healthy Plate. Your body needs food from each of them. Each food group has a different function. Let us find out what they are.

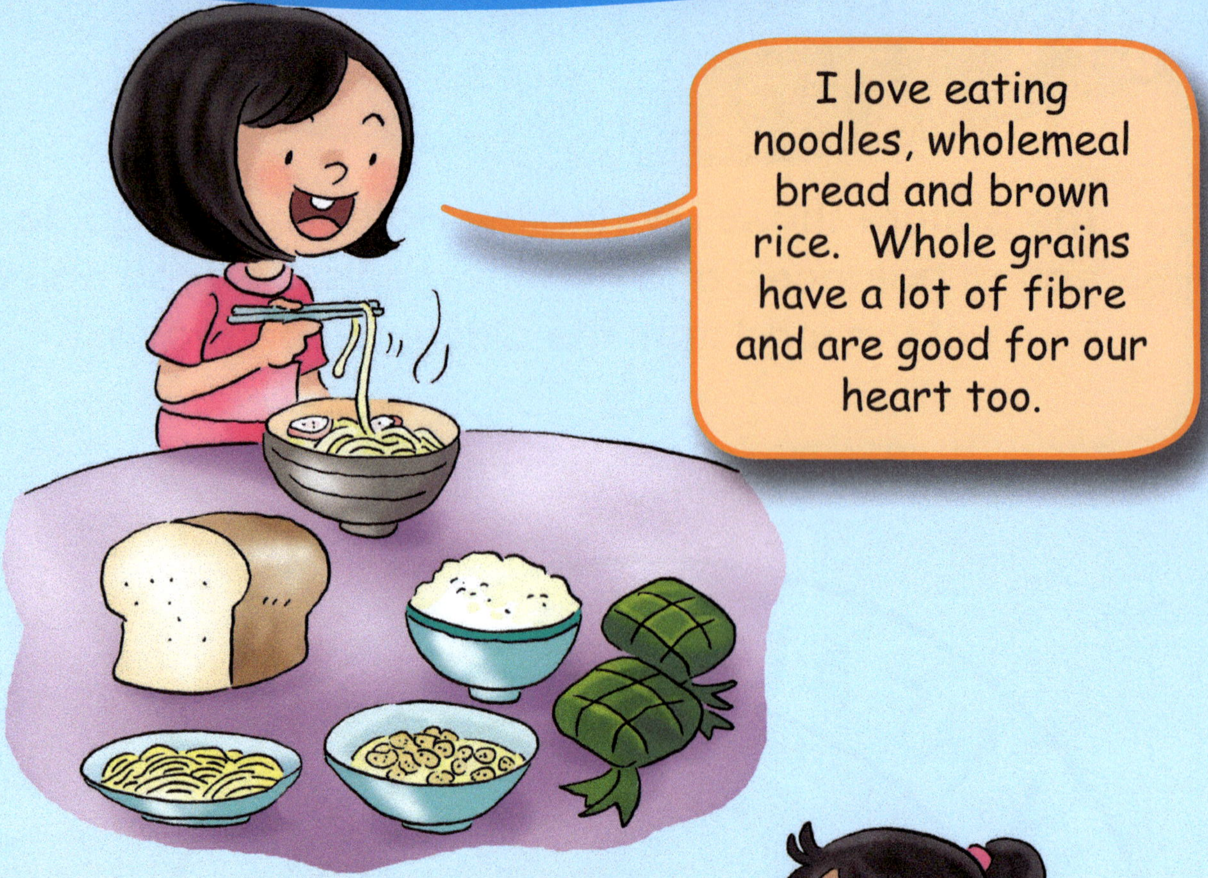

> I love eating noodles, wholemeal bread and brown rice. Whole grains have a lot of fibre and are good for our heart too.

> I love fruit and vegetables. They have lots of water, vitamins, minerals and fibre. They are important for healthy living.

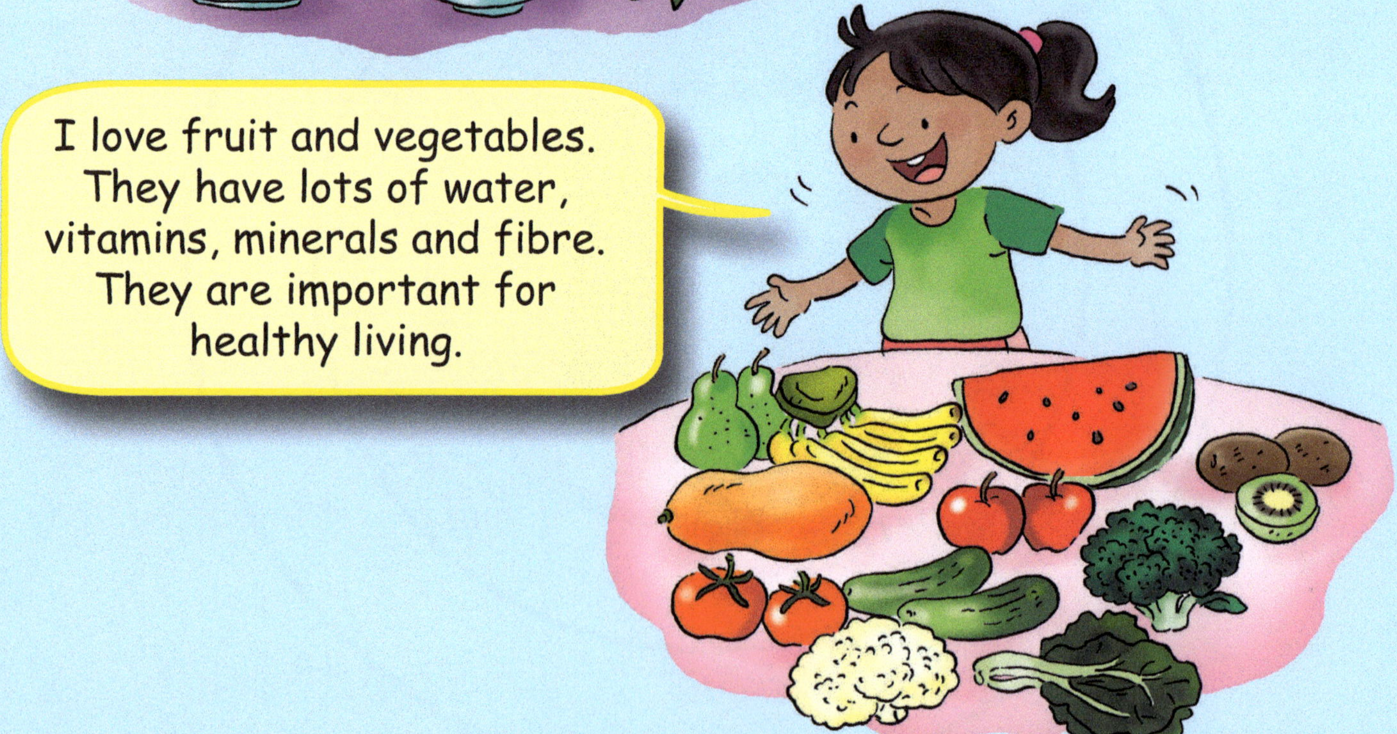

What about water? It is important to drink lots of water daily especially on a hot day and after strenuous sport or exercise.

Two of my favourite dishes are fish and chicken. You can find protein and fat in meat and fish. Protein helps us grow. Fat gives us energy and makes food tasty. Fish and tofu are healthier food items that contain protein.

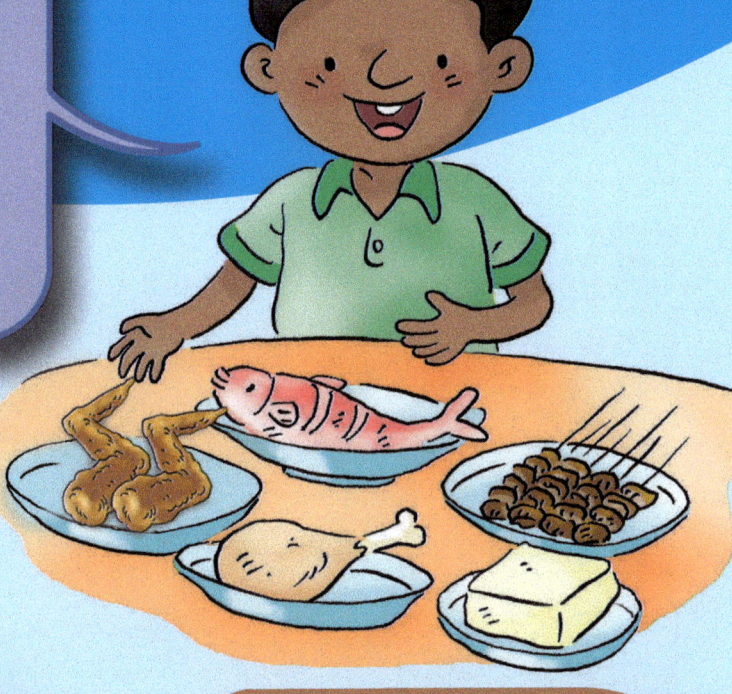

I have milk and some nuts and cereal every day. Milk belongs in the food group 'meat and others'. It contains calcium, which we need to build strong bones and teeth. Nuts are rich in protein. They contain healthy oils and are good for us.

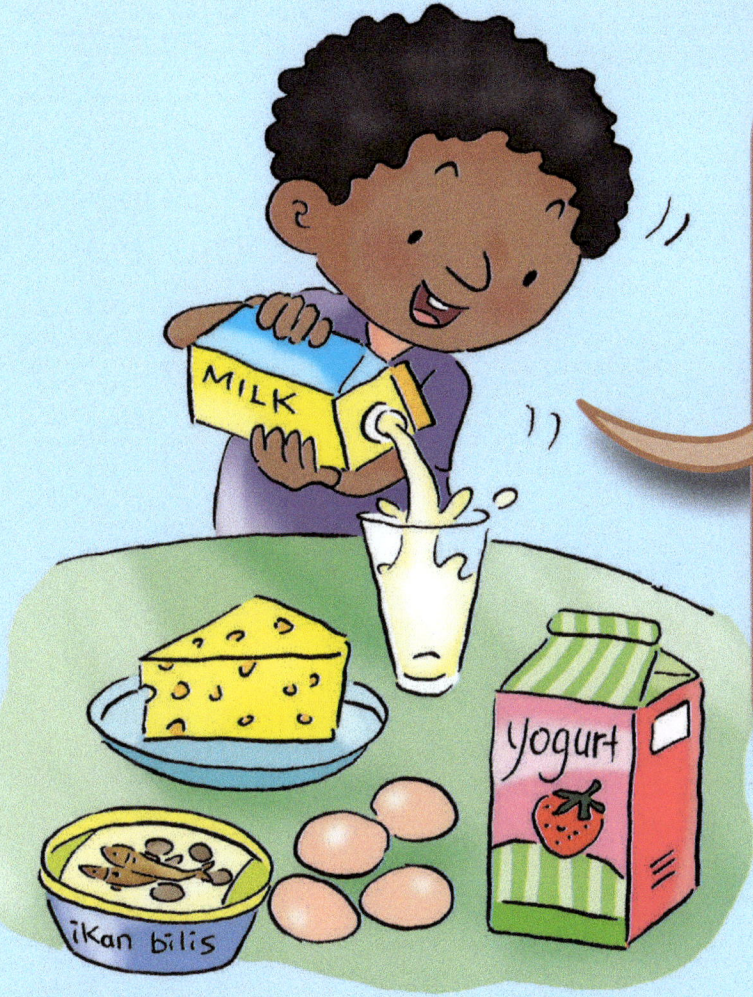

What about oil, salt and sugar? It can be unhealthy to have too much of them or take them too often. Your body does not need large amounts of these.

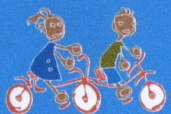 **Draw lines to match the food items to the correct food groups.**

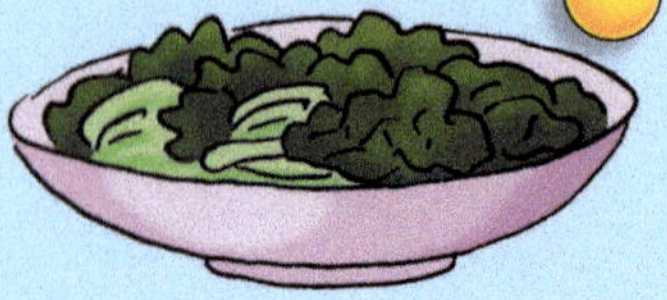

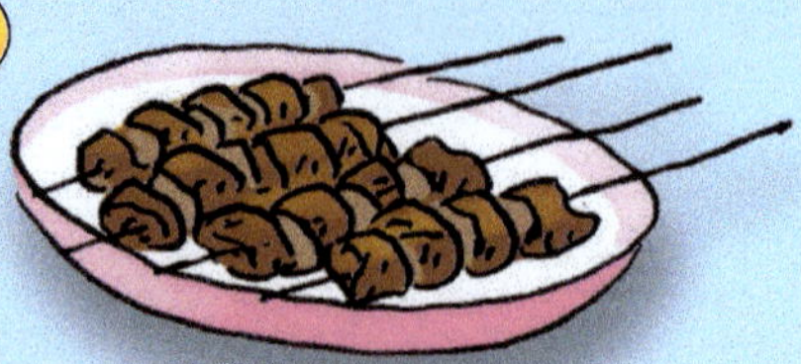

Vegetables

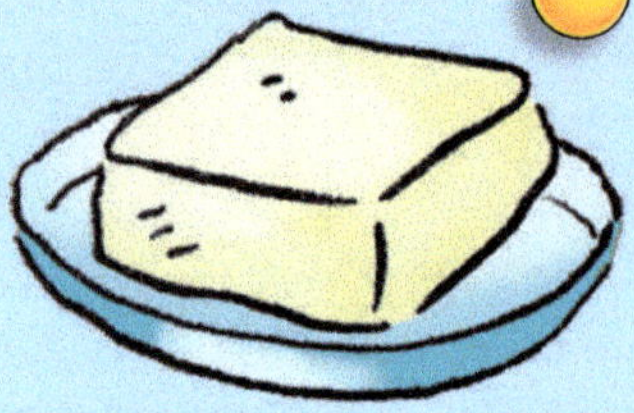

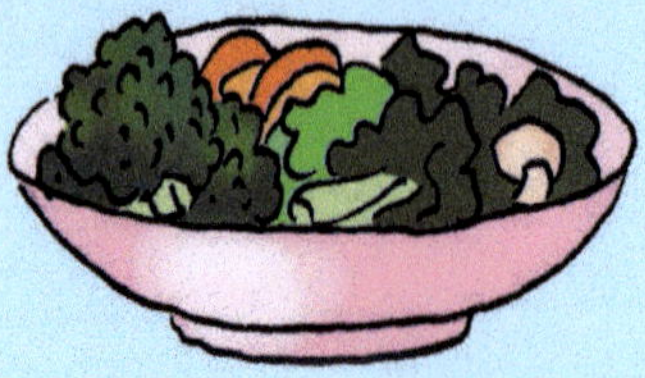

Meat and others

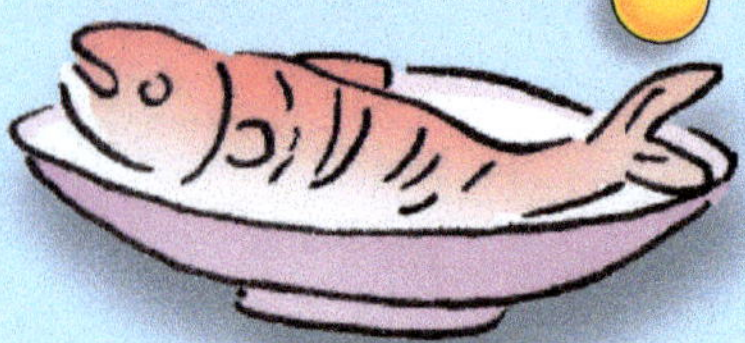

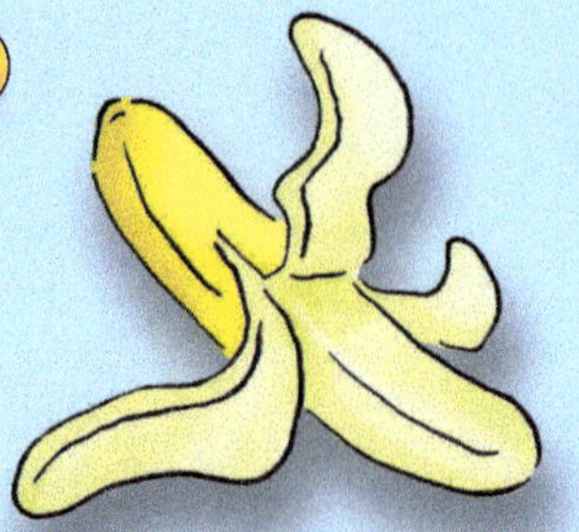

Whole grains

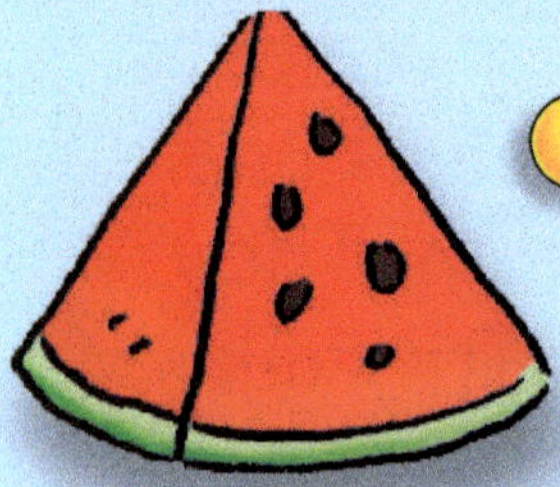

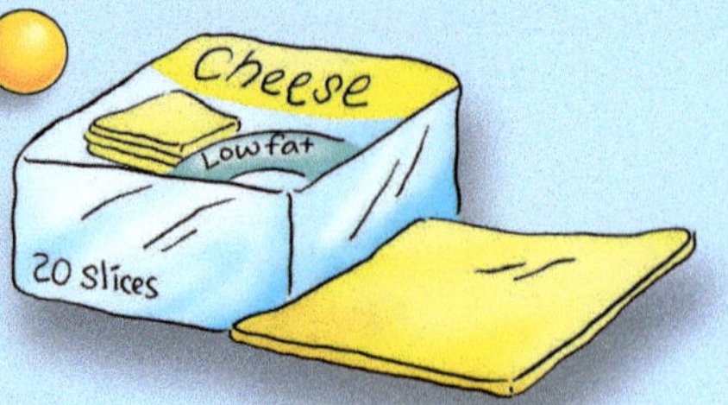

Fruit

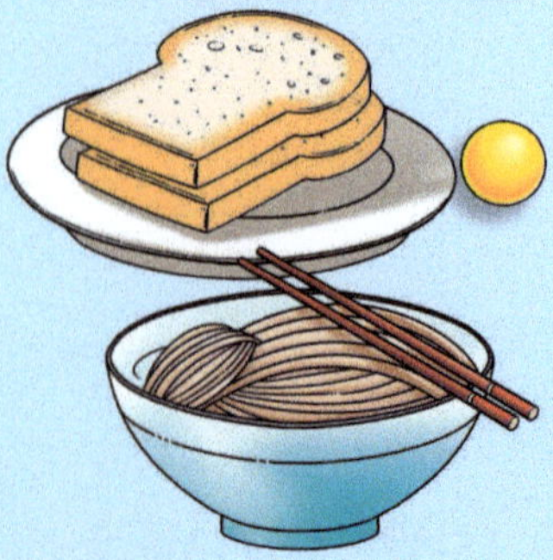

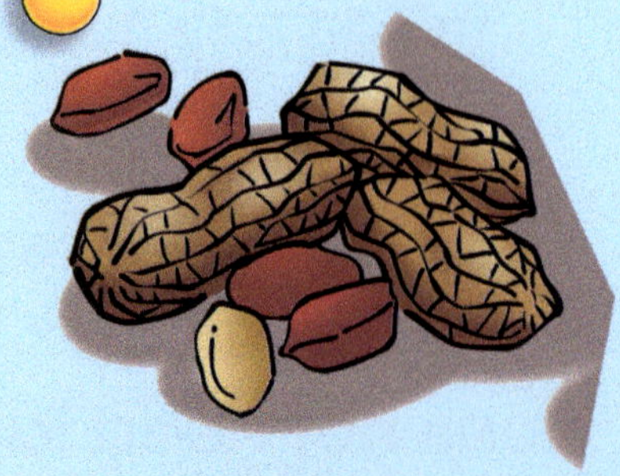

Name: Class: Date: Lesson 3

Food Detective

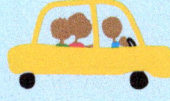

Now that you have learnt about My Healthy Plate, it is time for some detective work!

1. Look at the pictures below. Circle the food and drinks that are sold in your canteen every day.

- water
- milk
- juice
- rice with two dishes
- chicken rice
- fried noodles
- vegetables
- porridge
- noodle soup
- nasi lemak
- mee siam
- roti prata with curry
- sandwich
- banana
- papaya
- pineapple
- watermelon
- potato chips
- cake
- ice cream
- mung bean dessert

Learning Objectives: Pupils will be able to identify the different types of food for growth and health, and make healthy food choices to obtain and maintain healthy growth.

2. Visit your school canteen and look at the food for sale. Which food groups do they belong to?
List three items in each of the food groups below.

Fruit
_____
_____

Vegetables
_____
_____

Meat and Others
_____
_____
_____

Whole Grains
_____
_____
_____

Are there food items from My Healthy Plate that are not easy to find in your school canteen? Name **three** that you would like to have in your canteen (e.g. pasta, nuts, plain buns....)
_____
_____
_____

Name: Class: Date: Lesson 4

Am I Eating Right?

A healthy meal is one that contains a variety of food from the different food groups. It is also eaten with a drink such as water, milk or juice.

Look at the pictures below. Draw a  in the circle if the picture shows a healthy meal.

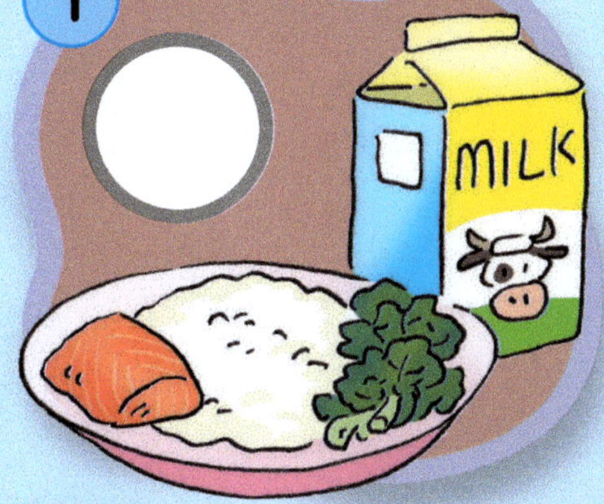

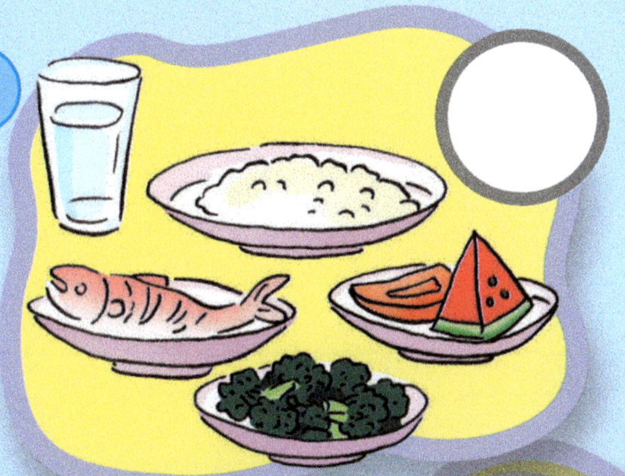

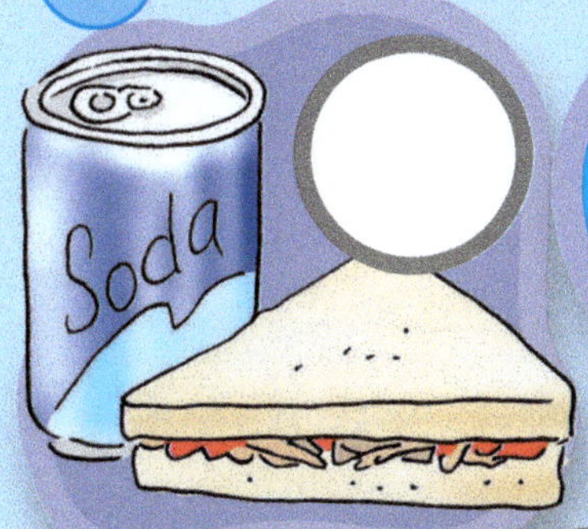

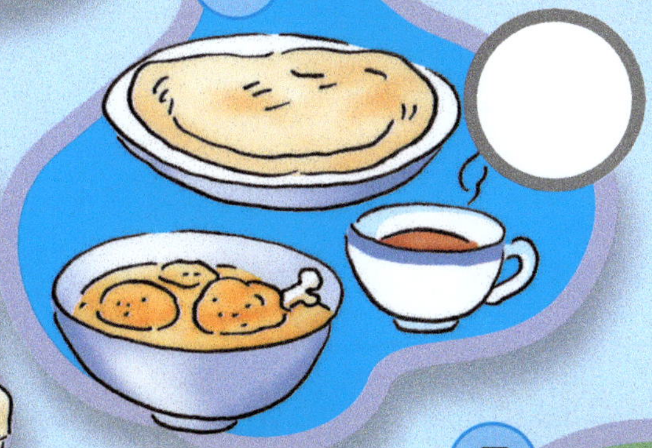

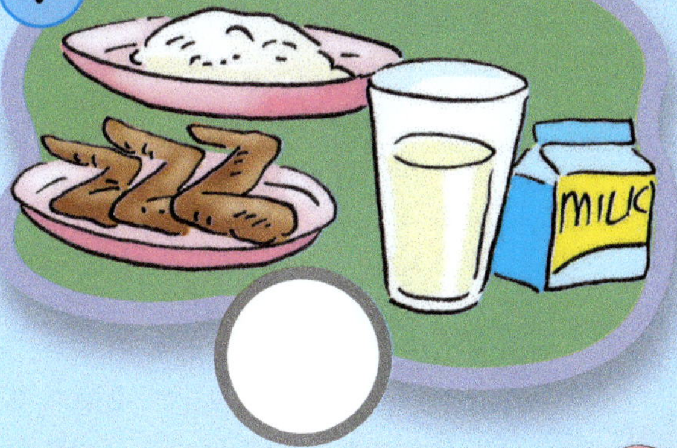

Learning Objectives: Pupils will be able to identify the different types of food for growth and health, and make healthy food choices to obtain and maintain healthy growth.

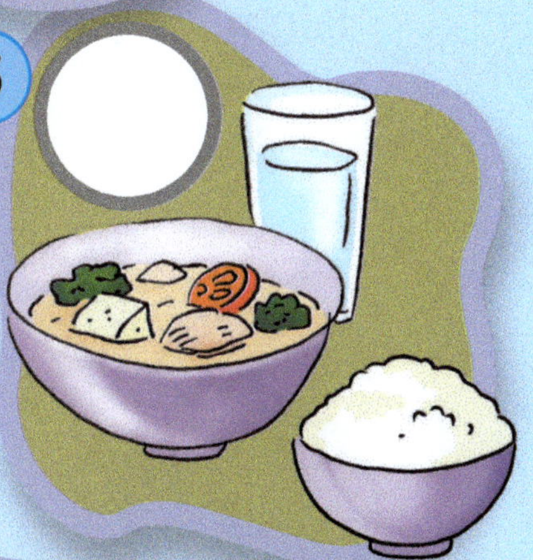

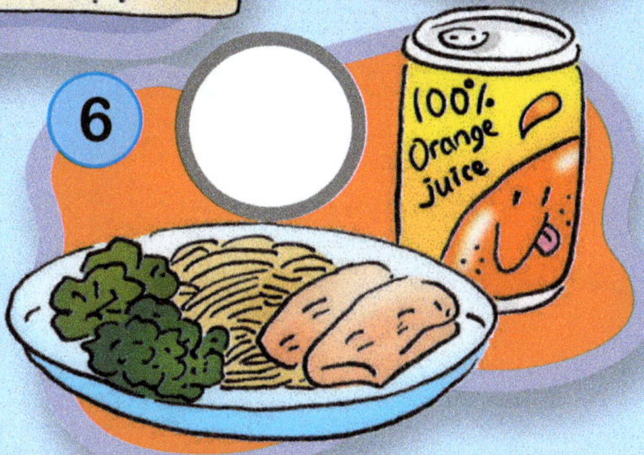

Think of what you had for breakfast, lunch and dinner yesterday. Write them in the spaces below.

Breakfast

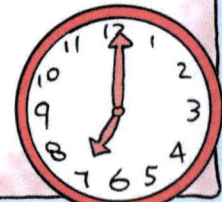

Lunch

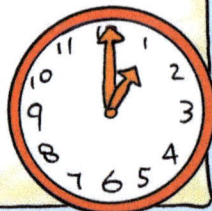

Dinner

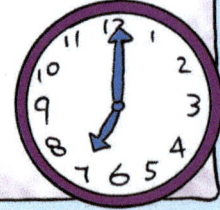

Was every meal you had a well-balanced one? Were you eating too much or too little of a type of food shown on My Healthy Plate? How can you make each meal more balanced?

Use My Healthy Plate to plan three healthy meals—breakfast, lunch and dinner.

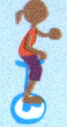

1. Look at the three plates. Write the name of a meal (breakfast, lunch or dinner) at the top of each plate.
2. Plan each meal and draw the food items in each section.
3. Cut along the outline of each plate.
4. Place the breakfast plate on top, followed by the lunch and dinner plates. Punch a hole through the three plates and tie a string through them.

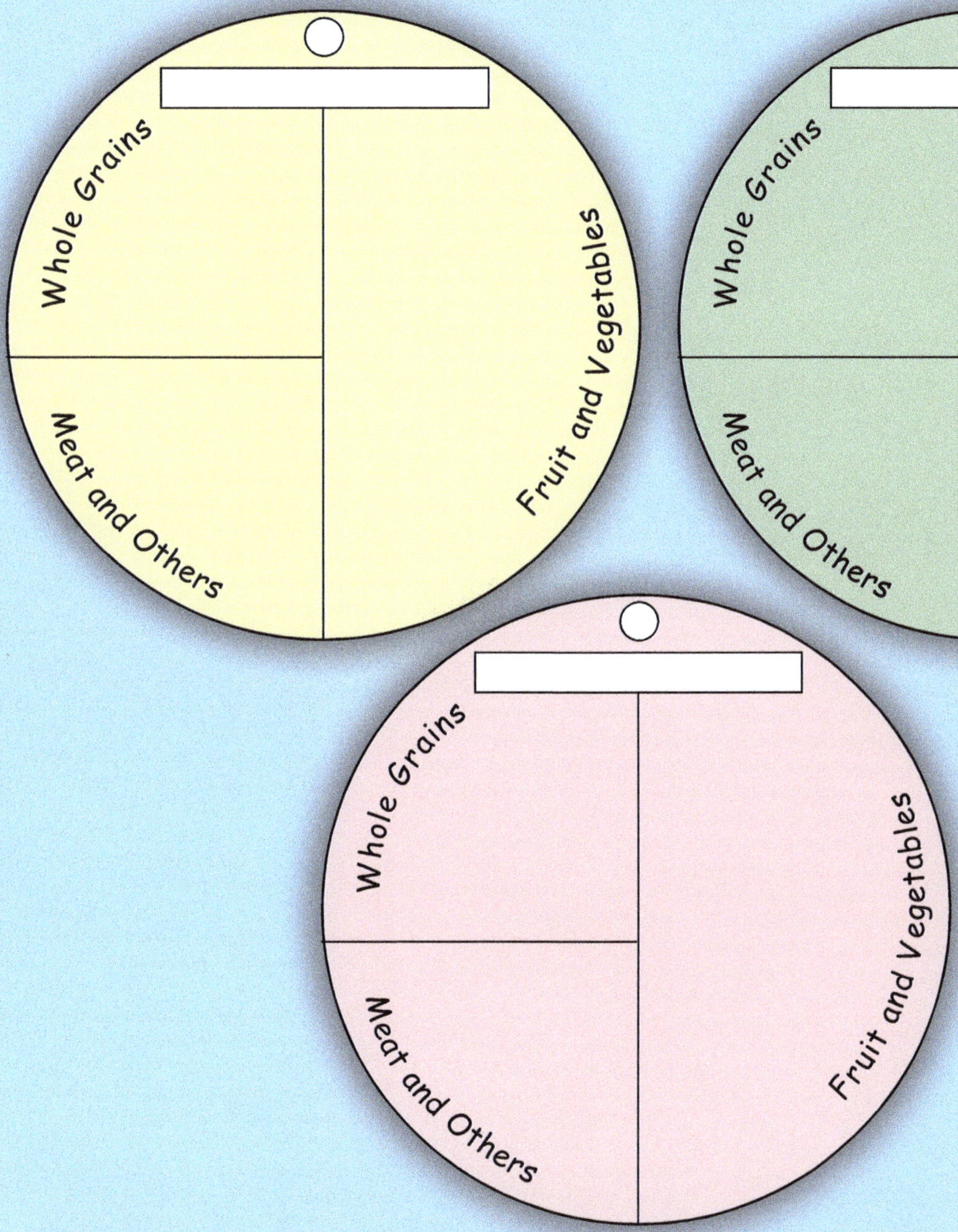

When you have finished, show your food plates to your partner.

This page is left blank for the cutting exercise on the previous page.

Name: _____ ____ ____

Lesson 5

Stay Active

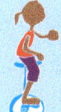 How much time should you spend doing the following every day?

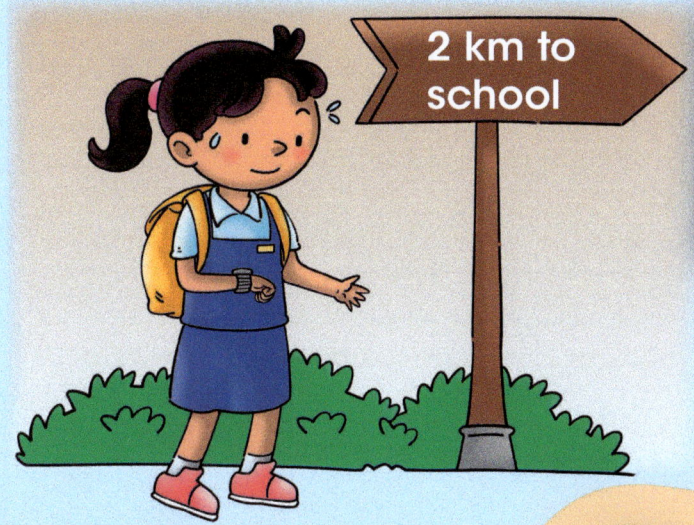

Working at something that uses a lot of energy or walking long distances.

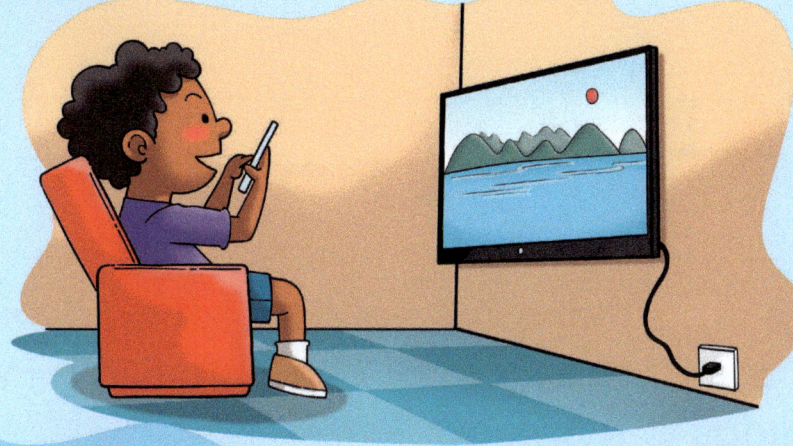

Sitting down to watch TV or use the computer or mobile phone.

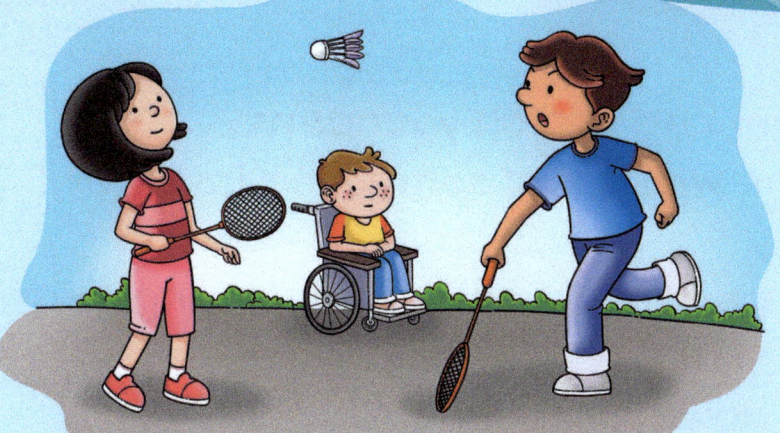

Spending time outdoors.

Learning Objectives: Pupils will be able to establish daily habits for caring for their bodies to maintain and improve health and prevent illness.

Do you move your body enough? To stay healthy, you should avoid sitting down all day. The time you spend on moderate-to-vigorous physical activities should add up to at least **60** minutes every day.

 What are "moderate-to-vigorous physical activities"? List five such activities you can do daily.

1. Help with the housework.
2.
3.
4.
5.

Do not sit for too long. After sitting down for about **30** minutes, move about for about three to five minutes. These are the things you can do:

- ✔ Stand up, walk about and stretch your arms.
- ✔ Try looking out of the window at something far away.
- ✔ Get a drink.
- ✔ See what the other people around you are doing.

Avoid the habit of sitting down all the time.

moderate-to-vigorous physical activities: when you do these activities, you will be breathing harder and faster. You will still be able to talk but you will find it difficult to sing.

Name: Class: Date: Lesson 6

A Dip In The Pool

Follow the story in the comic strip below.

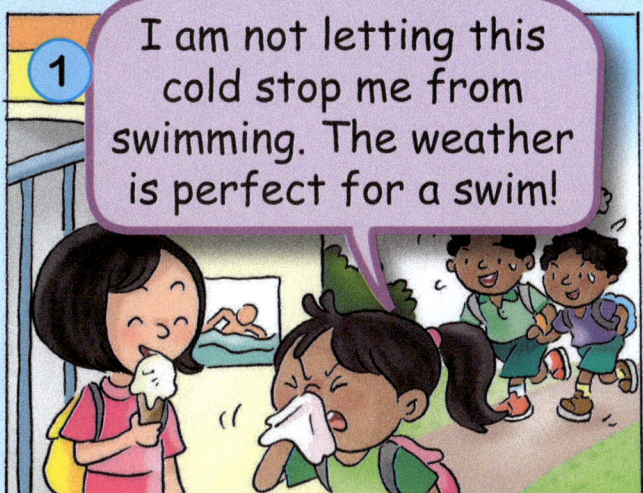

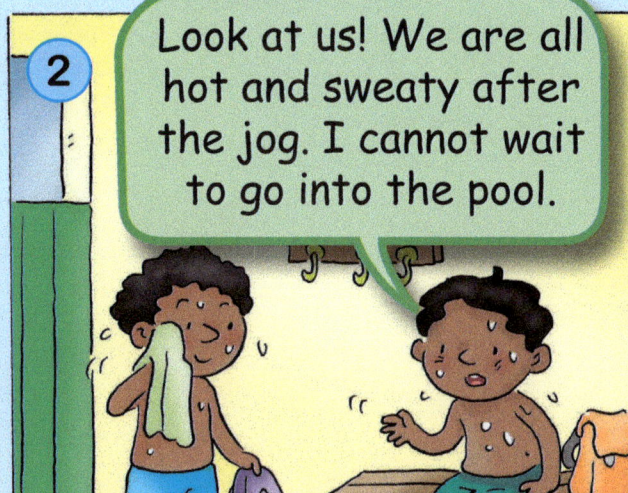

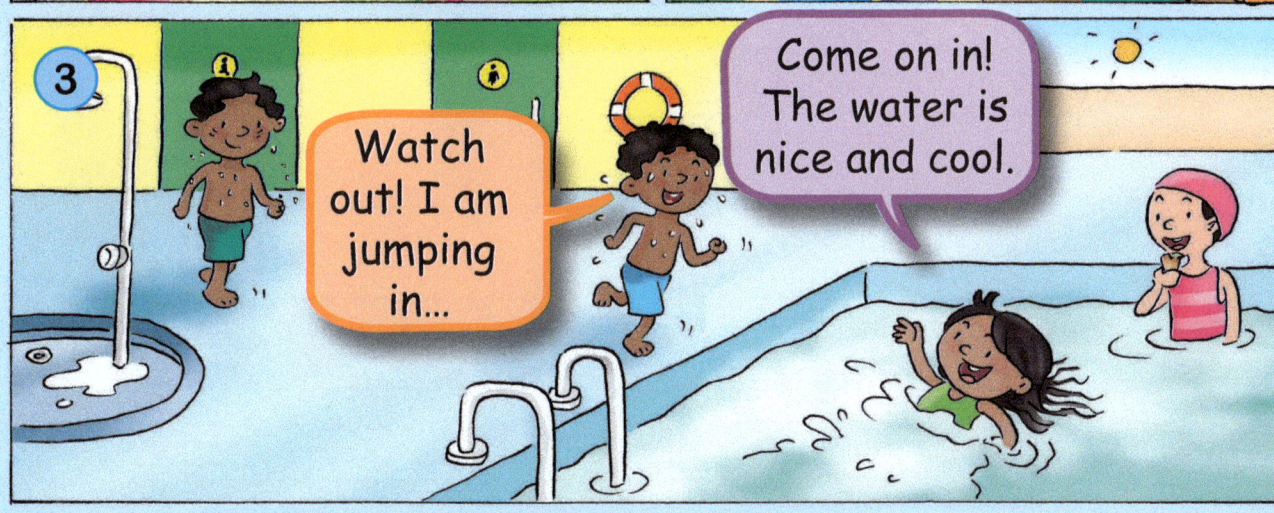

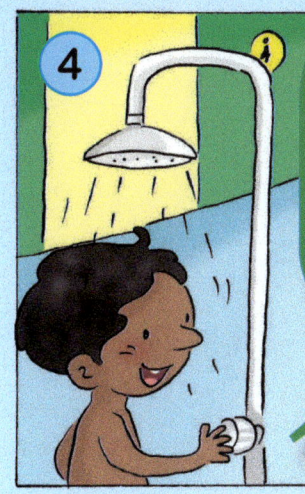

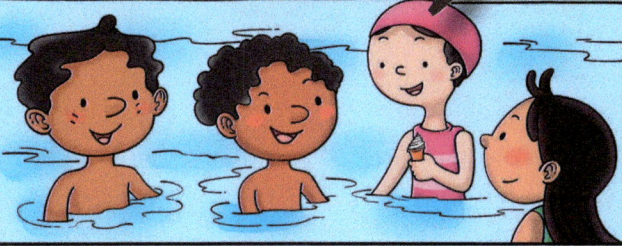

Learning Objective: Pupils will be able to establish daily habits for caring for their bodies in order to maintain or improve health and prevent illnesses.

Look at the comic strip again. Eileen, Tawan and Ajit did five things that they should not have done.

Identify their mistakes and describe what they should have done in the space below.

Name: Class: Date: Lesson 7

Should Lam Accept The Offer?

Poor Lam! He has lost his backpack and does not have the things for camping. The other superfriends offer him some items. Should Lam accept them?

Listen carefully as your teacher reads. Decide whether Lam should accept the items from his friends. Circle 'Y' for yes, and 'N' for no.

1. Should Lam accept Harold's offer? Y / N
2. Should Lam accept Haris's offer? Y / N
3. Should Lam accept Ajit's offer? Y / N
4. Should Lam accept Tawan's offer? Y / N
5. Should Lam accept Eileen's offer? Y / N
6. Should Lam accept Harold's second offer? Y / N
7. Should Lam accept Haris's second offer? Y / N
8. Should Lam accept Ajit's second offer? Y / N

Learning Objective: Pupils will be able to establish daily habits for caring for their bodies in order to maintain or improve health and prevent illnesses.

Just like you should shower every day, you should also change your clothes daily. This will help you keep clean. For hygiene reasons, you should not share some things with others.

 Circle the items you should change every day. Cross out the items you should not share with others.

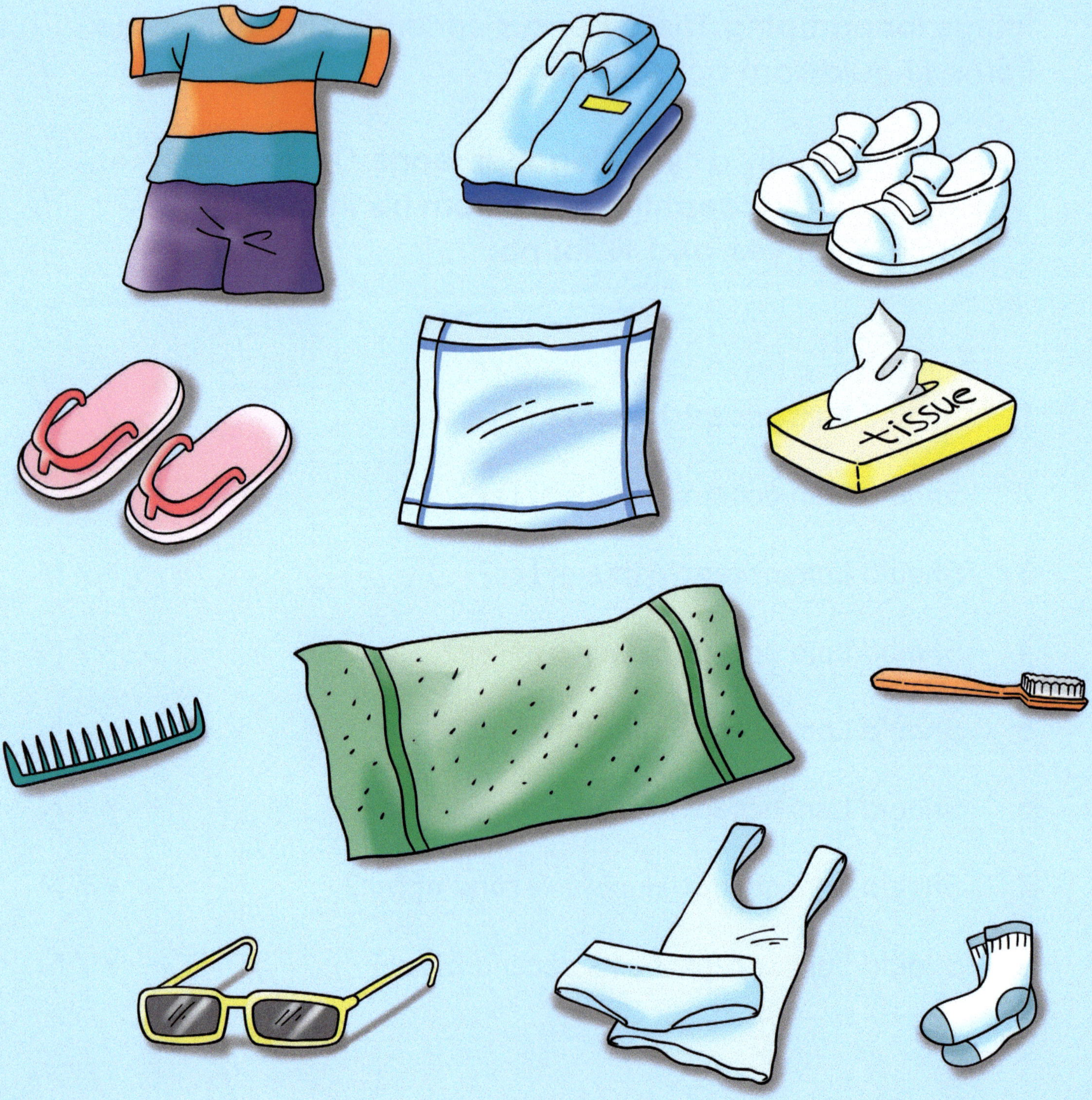

Name: Class: Date: Lesson 8

Look At Our Posters

It is important to keep clean because being clean keeps germs away. Germs can cause diseases and make us ill.

Look at the posters the superfriends have made. Which of them describe good hygiene practices? Circle the posters.

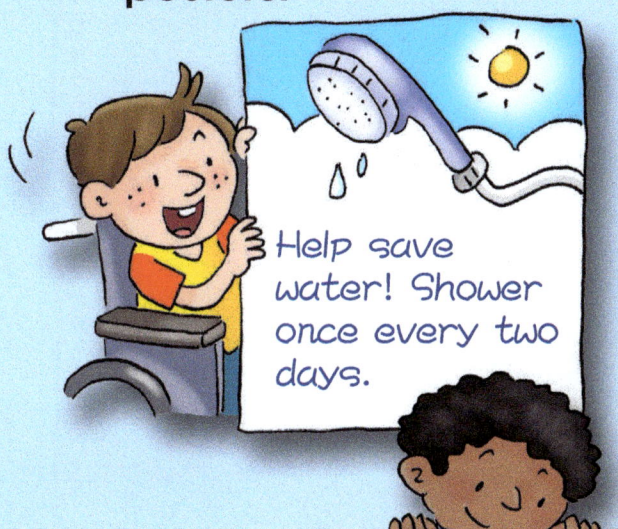
Help save water! Shower once every two days.

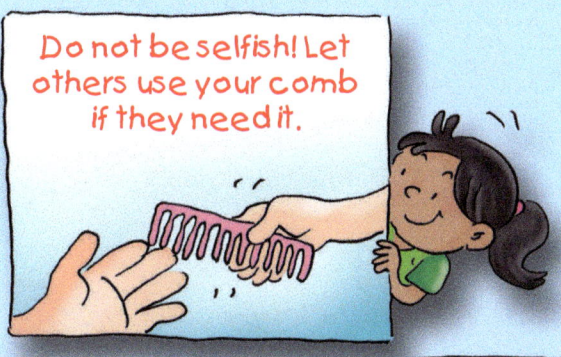
Do not be selfish! Let others use your comb if they need it.

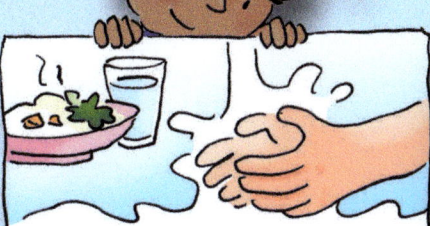
Washing your hands is important, especially before meals.

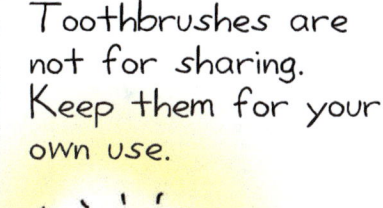
Toothbrushes are not for sharing. Keep them for your own use.

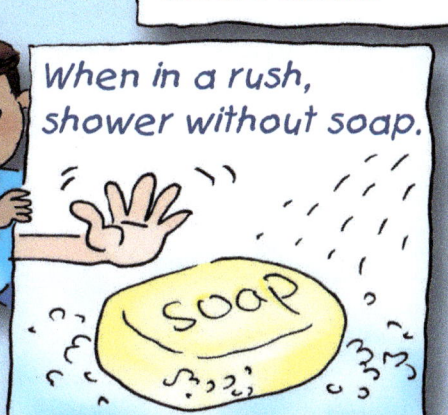
When in a rush, shower without soap.

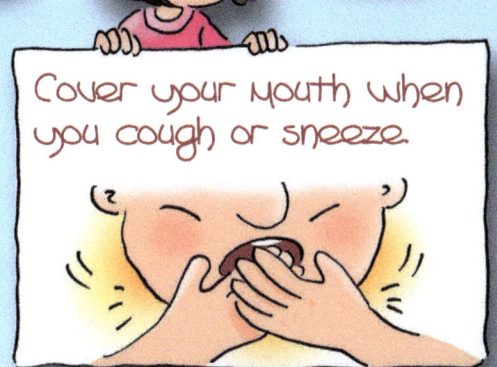
Cover your mouth when you cough or sneeze.

Learning Objective: Pupils will be able to establish daily habits for caring for their bodies in order to maintain or improve health and prevent illnesses.

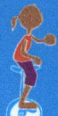 **Make your own poster about a good hygiene practice in the space below. Use it to remind yourself about how you can keep clean.**

Name: Class: Date:

Lessons 9

Give Your Eyes A Break

Look at the picture below. Circle the superfriends who are hurting their eyes.

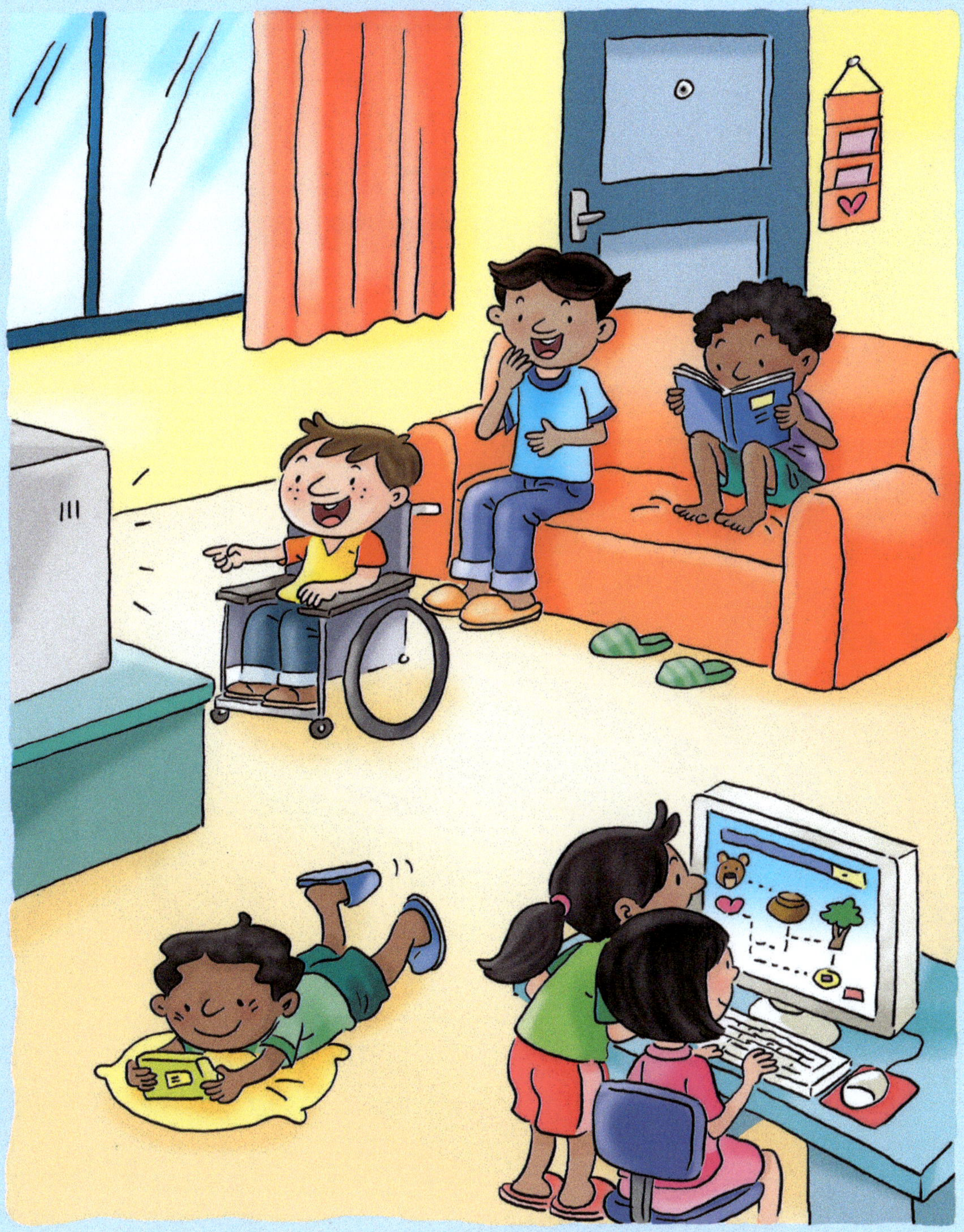

Learning Objective: Pupils will be able to recognise that the eyes need proper care and rest for good vision.

From the time you wake up to the time you fall asleep, your eyes work very hard for you. They help you to read, watch television, use your computer and do many other things.

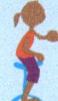 How can you take care of your eyes? Listen carefully as your teacher reads and fill in the blanks.

Make sure there is enough l_____ so that you will not strain your eyes.

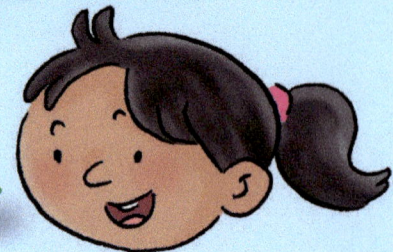

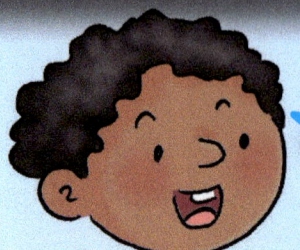

When you watch television, sit at least t__ metres away from the television screen.

Also, make sure the television screen is b_____ or at your eye level.

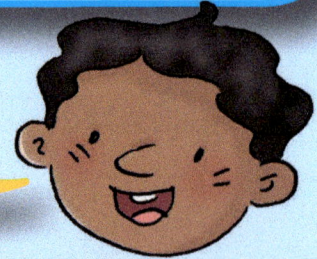

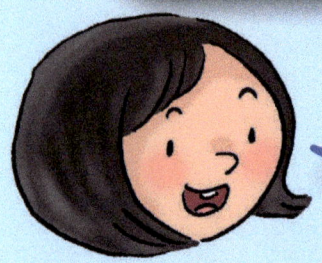

When you do any near work activity, give your eyes a break every t_____ to f_____ minutes for at least t_____ to f____ minutes. Look at an object far away.

What is a near work activity?

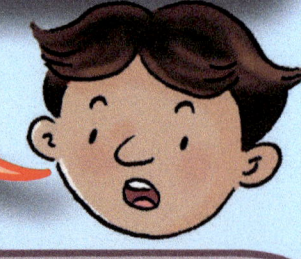

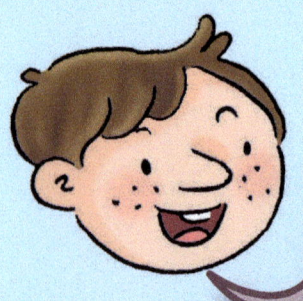

It is an activity that you do within an arm's length. Examples of near work activities are r_____, writing, using the c_____, and watching t_____.

Name: Class: Date: Lessons 10

Something To To Chew On

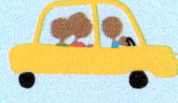

Hidden in the puzzle below are six words describing food which are good for our teeth and things which help us take care of them.

The words are written horizontally, vertically and diagonally. Circle them. Then write them in the box below.

T	L	E	T	M	E	A	L	S	Y
K	O	S	O	O	I	L	I	I	O
U	L	O	O	A	I	L	C	O	G
Z	L	G	T	H	O	E	K	L	U
O	I	T	H	H	A	M	I	K	R
Y	P	I	P	W	B	S	W	E	T
G	O	L	A	U	S	R	L	E	S
A	P	B	S	T	I	E	U	A	I
S	S	E	T	H	F	L	O	S	S
C	H	E	E	S	E	R	A	S	H

Learning Objective: Pupils will be able to recognise the importance of developing good oral hygiene habits to ensure that the teeth are healthy and well maintained.

25

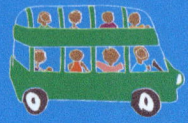

Milk, cheese and green leafy vegetables are good for the teeth because they are high in calcium. Calcium helps keep your bones and teeth strong. Examples of calcium-rich foods are shown below.

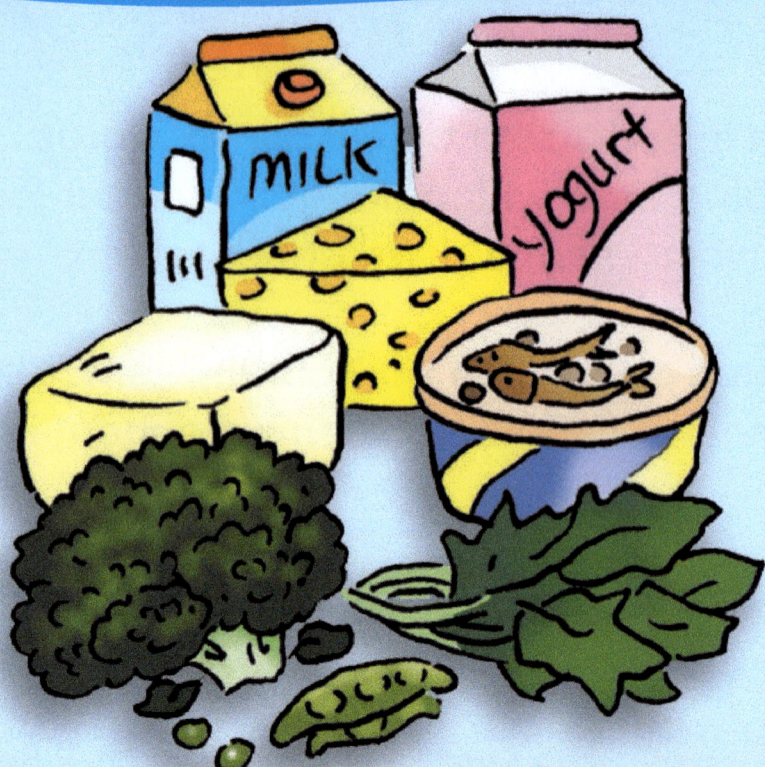

Milk, cheese, green leafy vegetables, *ikan bilis* (anchovies), beancurd and yogurt all contain calcium.

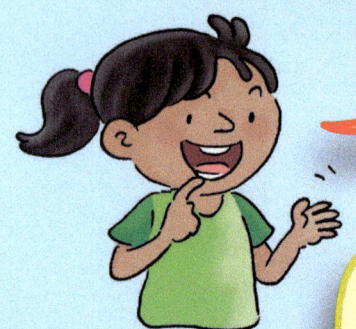

So, remember to take care of your teeth. Brush with some toothpaste after meals.

Make sure you brush and floss correctly. Clean your tongue gently with a toothbrush or a tongue scraper.

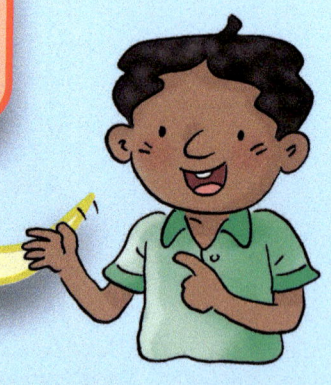

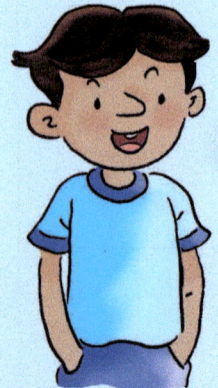

Eat calcium-rich foods …

… and visit your dentist once every six months.

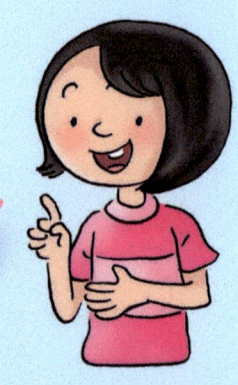

Environment And Your Health

In this section, you will learn:

- how diseases can spread; and
- about dengue fever and how to prevent it.

A Picnic

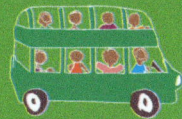

Follow the story in the comic strip below. What do you think happened the day after the picnic?

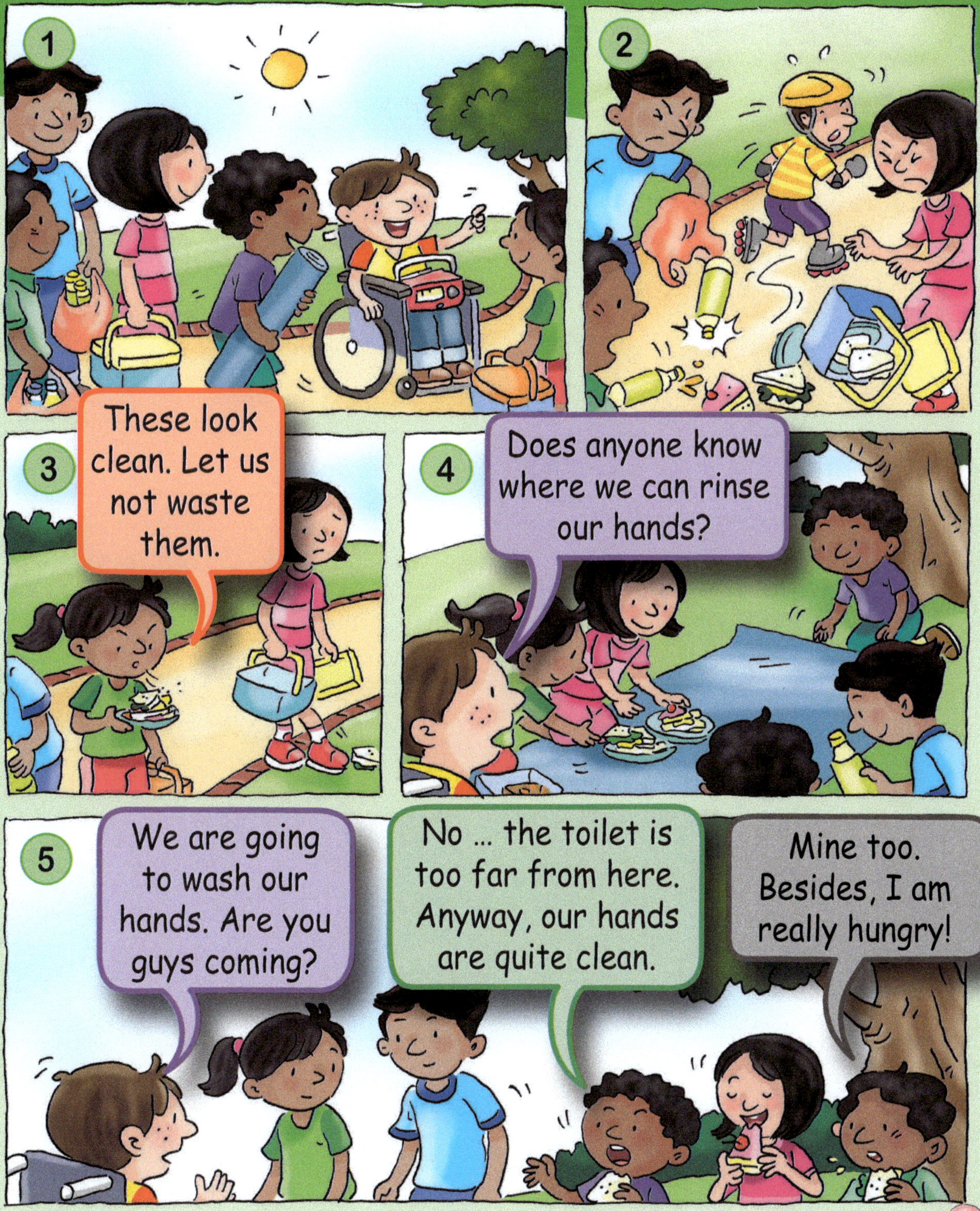

Contaminated food and drinks can spread diseases and make you ill. That is why you must practise good hygiene when you prepare food and drinks. You must also wash your hands before you eat or drink.

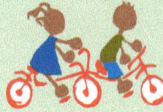 Look at the pictures below. What do you think Tawan and Ajit should have said to Eileen and Harold?

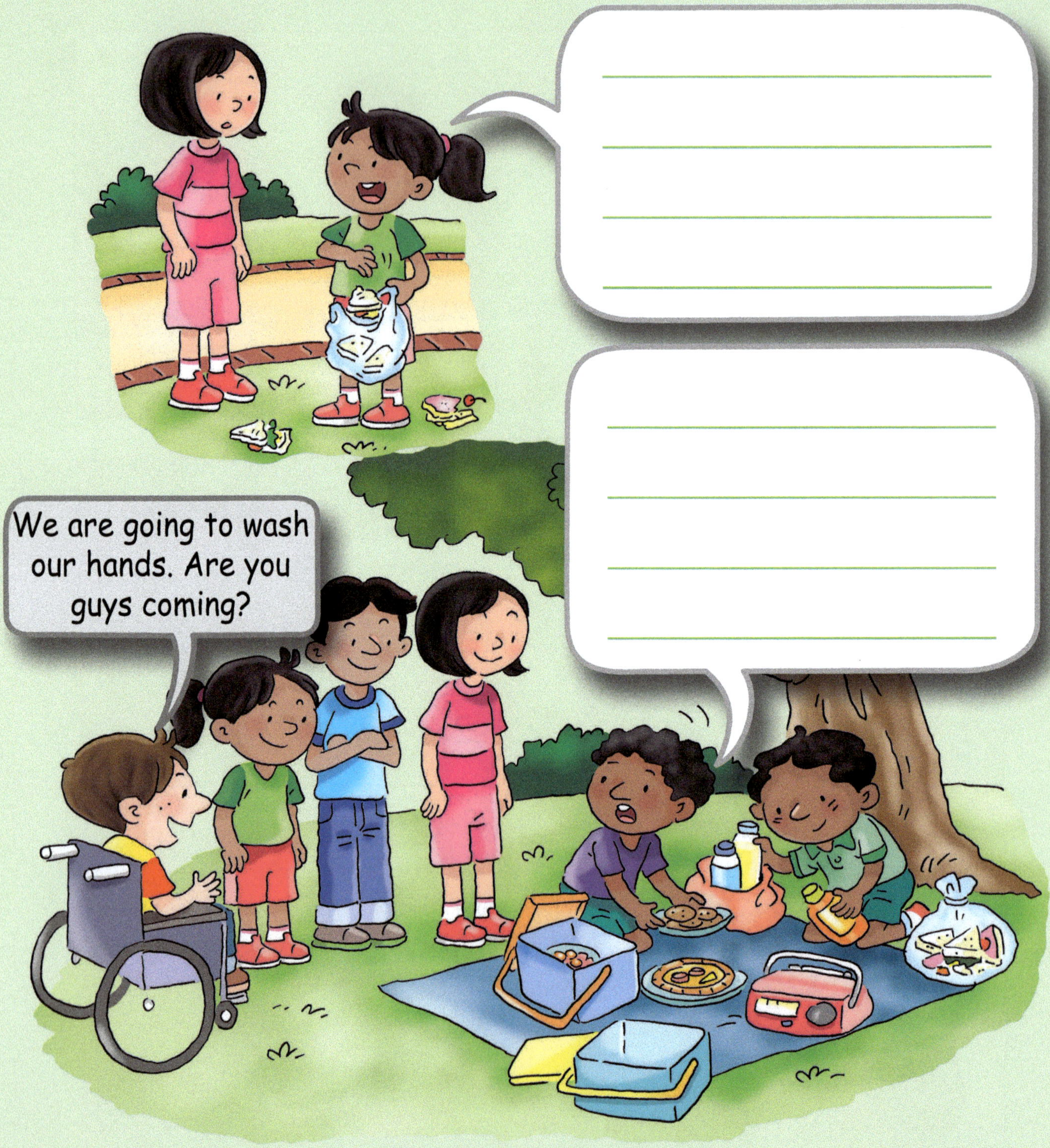

contaminated: dirtied or spoilt.

Name: Class: Date: Lesson 2

Trouble In The Kitchen

There are ten problems related to safety and hygiene in the picture below. Identify and circle them. Then complete the exercise on the next page.

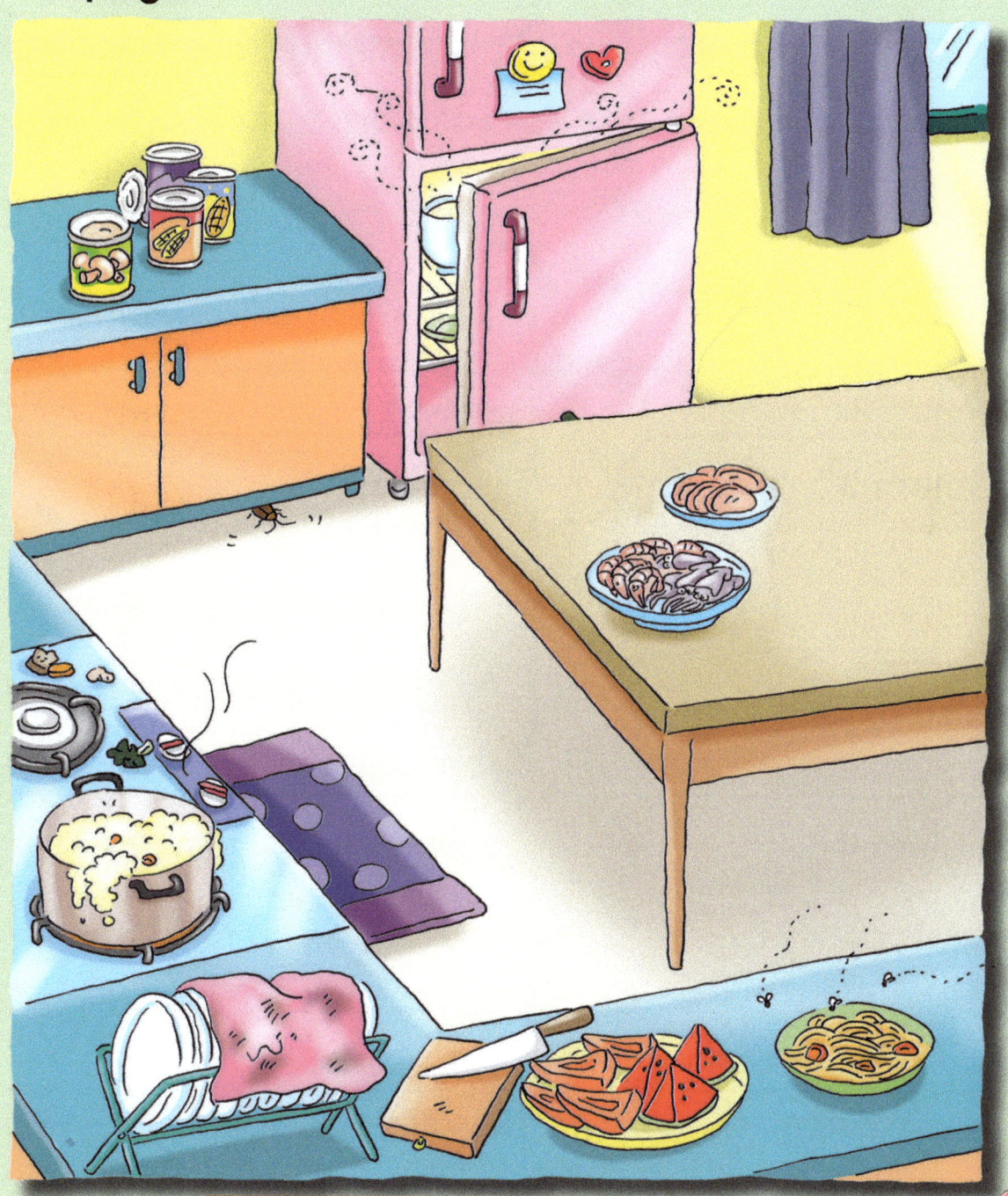

Learning Objective: Pupils will be able to recognise that an unclean environment is a risk to healthy living for everyone.

31

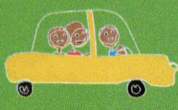

Choose any four problems that you have identified and think of a solution for each of them. Describe the problems and their solutions in the spaces provided.

Problem 1

Solution

Problem 2

Solution

Problem 3

Solution

Problem 4

Solution

Name: Class: Date: Lesson 3

Kitchen Hygiene

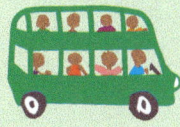

The superfriends are taking part in a kitchen hygiene cooking competition. The pictures below show what they are preparing.

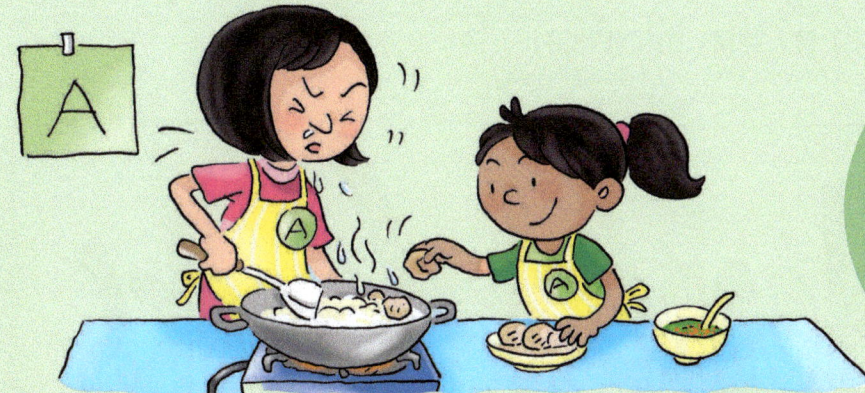

Tawan and Eileen are preparing chicken fried rice.

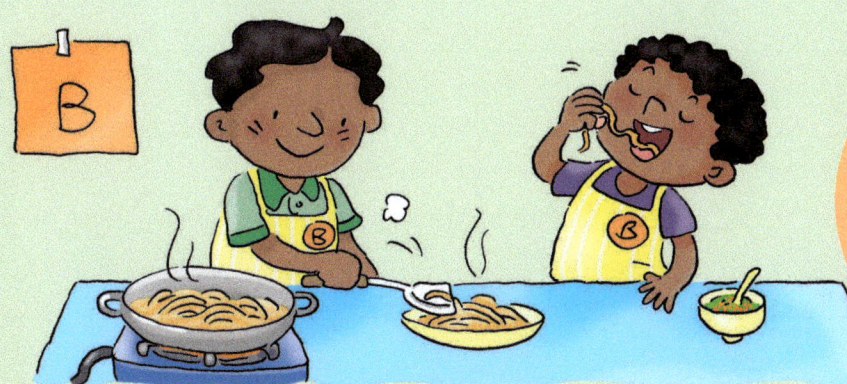

Ajit and Haris are frying some noodles.

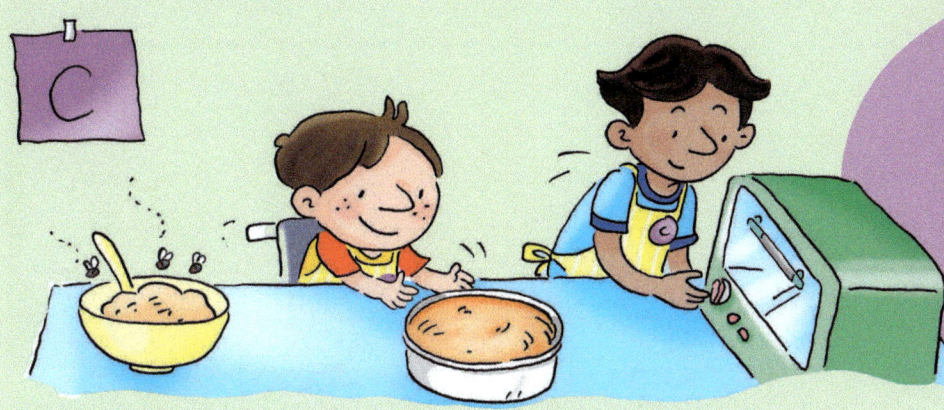

Harold and Lam are baking a cake.

Learning Objective: Pupils will be able to recognise that an unclean environment is a risk to healthy living for everyone.

It's time for the results! Oh dear, the judges do not look very impressed. What do you think they wrote on their comment sheet below? Discuss with your partner and fill in the blanks.

Cleanest Cooks

Tawan and Eileen: _____

_____

_____

Ajit and Haris: _____

_____

_____

Harold and Lam: _____

_____

_____

Name: Class: Date:

Lessons 4 & 5

No More Mosquitoes

Follow the story in the comic strip below.

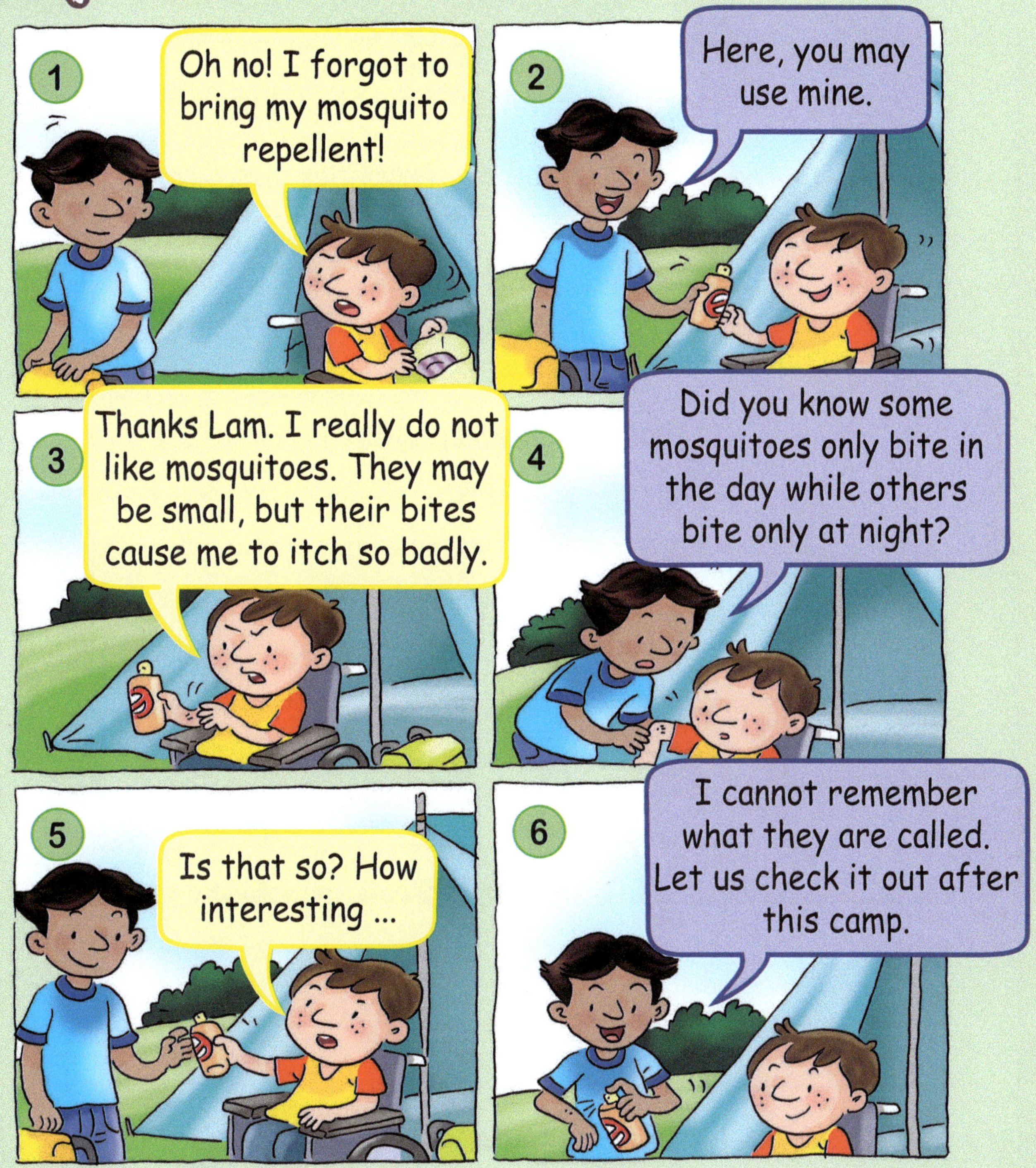

1. Oh no! I forgot to bring my mosquito repellent!

2. Here, you may use mine.

3. Thanks Lam. I really do not like mosquitoes. They may be small, but their bites cause me to itch so badly.

4. Did you know some mosquitoes only bite in the day while others bite only at night?

5. Is that so? How interesting ...

6. I cannot remember what they are called. Let us check it out after this camp.

 mosquito repellent: something that keeps mosquitoes away.

Learning Objective: Pupils will be able to recognise that an unclean environment is a risk to healthy living for everyone.

After the camp, Harold and Lam went to read up more about mosquitoes. They learnt that the Aedes mosquito mostly bites in the day whereas the Anopheles mosquito bites at night.

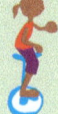 Harold and Lam decided to each prepare a report to share what they have learnt with the other superfriends. Help them complete their reports. Listen carefully as your teacher reads.

The Anopheles Mosquito by Harold

This is a photograph of the Anopheles mosquito.

(paste photograph here)

It bites only at _____. The Anopheles mosquito can cause _____ such as _____. When a person is ill with _____, he or she will have the following symptoms:

1. _____;

2. _____; and

3. _____.

Like all mosquitoes, the Anopheles mosquito breeds in _____ _____.

The Aedes Mosquito by Lam.

This is a photograph of the Aedes mosquito.

(paste photograph here)

It mostly bites in the _____. The Aedes mosquito can cause _____ such a _____ and _____. When a person is ill with _____ or _____, he or she will have the following symptoms:

1. _____;
2. _____; and
3. _____.

Like all mosquitoes, the Aedes mosquito breeds in _____ and _____.

Mosquitoes may be very small, but they can be dangerous. Learn to protect yourself from them!

Harold decided to find out more about the Aedes mosquito and what he can do to stop it from breeding. Look at what he learnt.

How can we stop the Aedes mosquito from breeding?

1. Change the water in all vases or bowls every other day.

2. Turn over all containers that store water.

3. Clear all drains and pipes to prevent water from collecting in them. If you live in a house, put BTI insecticides in the roof gutters every month.

4. Remove water from your flowerpots every two days.

5. Cover the bamboo pole holders when they are not used.

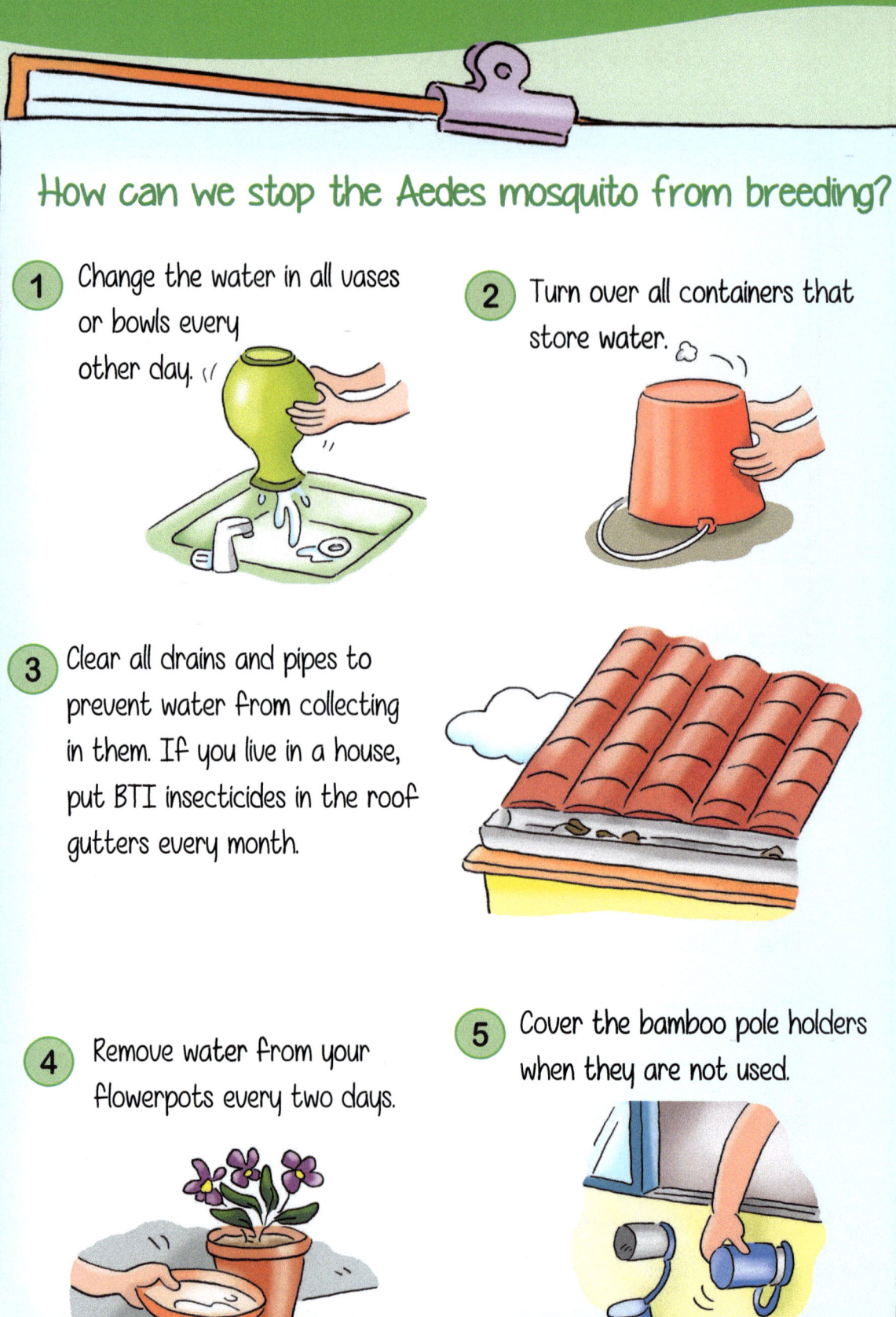

The countries in Southeast Asia are hot and wet. This makes it easy for the Aedes mosquitoes to breed. The female mosquito is the one which bites humans. It needs human blood so it can produce eggs. The female Aedes spreads diseases such as dengue and zika.

How does the Aedes mosquito spread dengue?

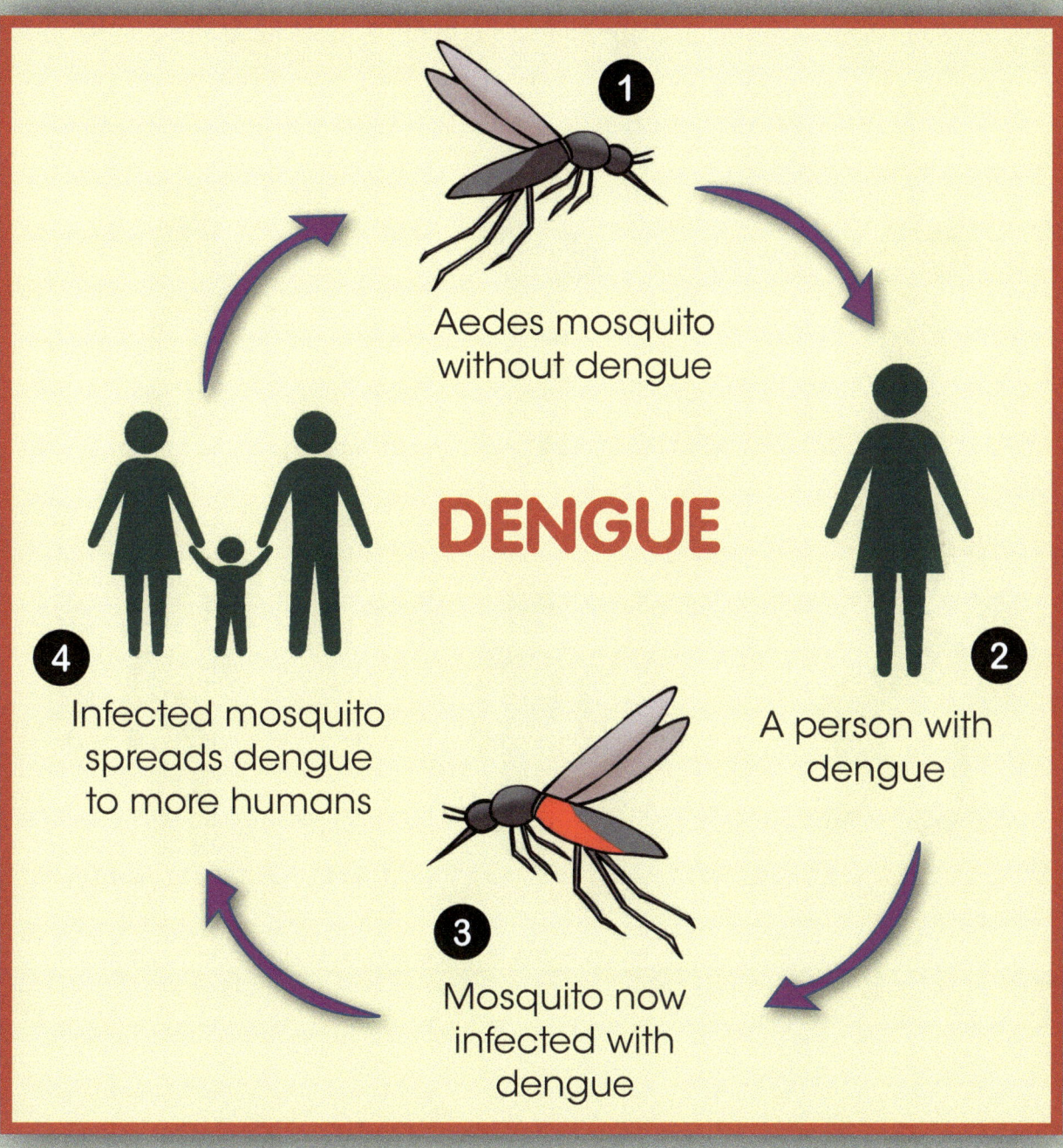

How would you know if you have dengue fever? Below are the symptoms of the illness. See a doctor immediately if you think you may be ill with dengue.

SYMPTOMS OF DENGUE

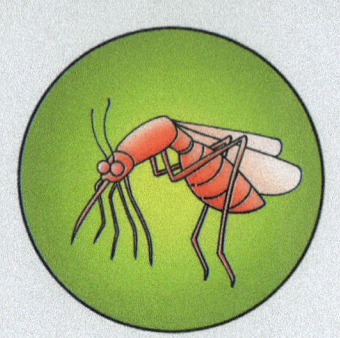

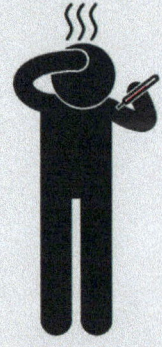

Sudden high fever

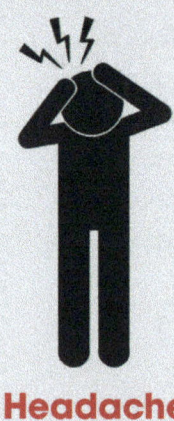

Headache

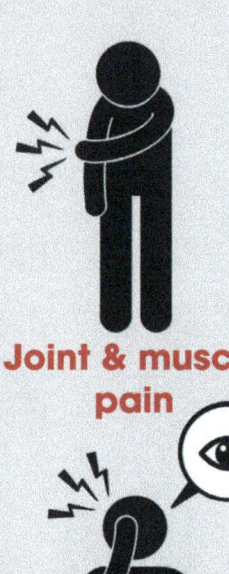

Joint & muscle pain

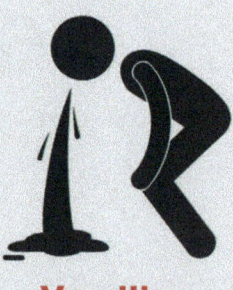

Vomiting

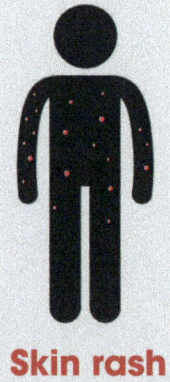

Skin rash

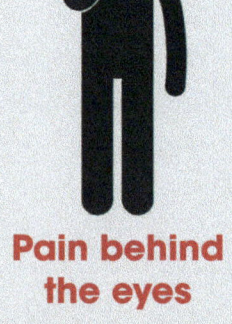

Pain behind the eyes

Emotional And Psychological Health

In this section, you will learn:

- some causes of conflicts and how to resolve them;
- how to recognise signs of low self-confidence; and
- how to be more confident of yourself.

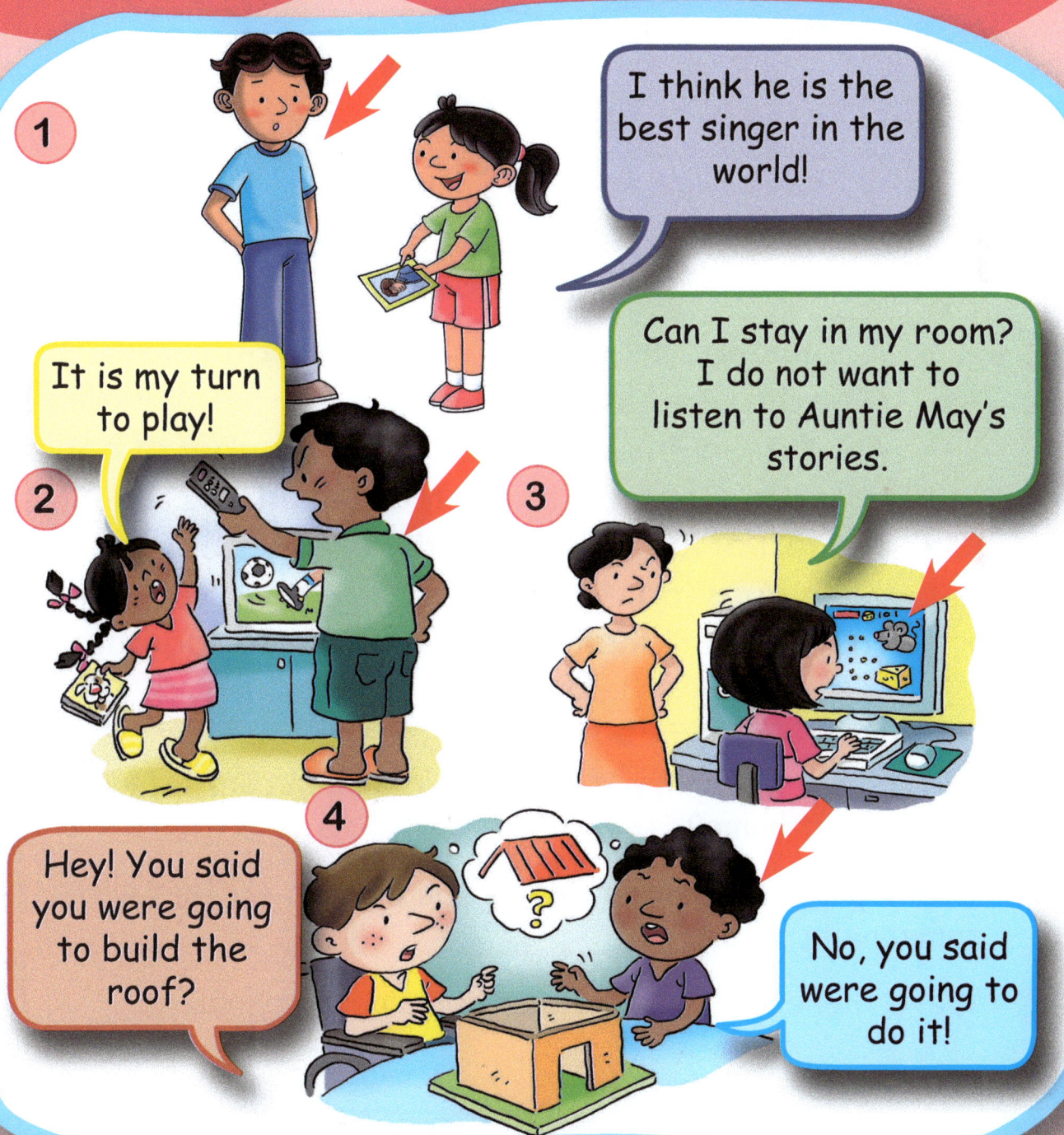

Have you ever felt like the superfriends on the previous page? You may not always agree with your family members or friends. But if you let them know, they may get angry with you.

When people do not agree with each other and they get angry, there will be a conflict. Conflicts can happen anywhere and at any time.

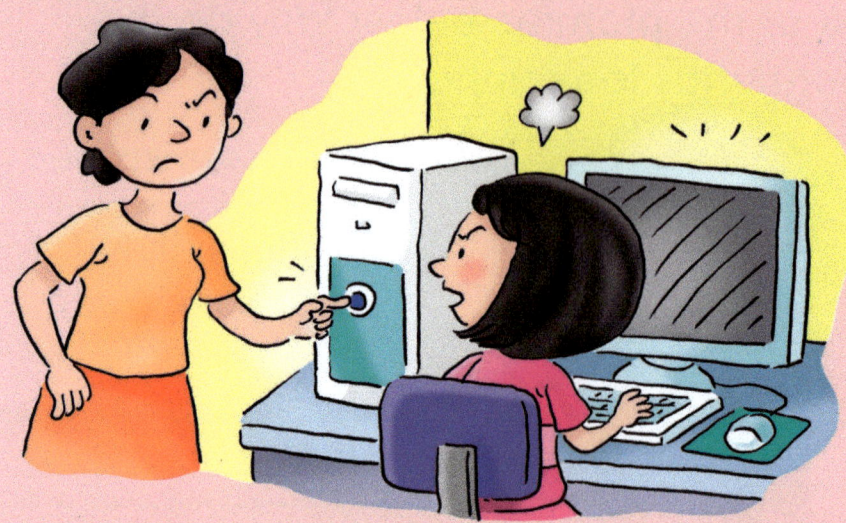

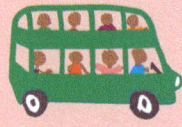

- A volunteer will ask the class three questions. (See the questions below.)
- Another volunteer will count the number of hands raised in response to each question.
- The rest of the class will write the number next to each question.
- The class will then answer Question 3 together.

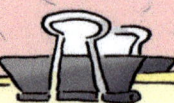

1. In the past week, how many of you were in conflict with someone at home? _____

2. In the past week, how many of you were in conflict with someone in school? _____

3. Were there more conflicts at home or in school?
   _____

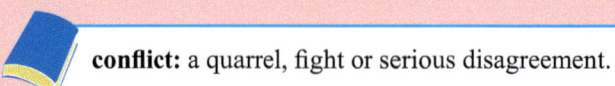

conflict: a quarrel, fight or serious disagreement.

| Name: | Class: | Date: | Lesson 2 |

Would You Get Angry?

Listen carefully as your teacher reads. Do you think there will be a conflict? Circle 'Y' for yes and 'N' for no.

1. Tawan and her grandma   Y / N

2. Tawan and Eileen   Y / N

3. Tawan and Ajit   Y / N

4. Tawan and Harold   Y / N

5. Tawan and Haris   Y / N

6. Tawan and Lam   Y / N

7. Eileen and Tawan   Y / N

8. Ajit and Tawan   Y / N

Learning Objective: Pupils will be able to understand how conflicts with others may be avoided or resolved.

Conflicts may happen when you do not understand a person. You may not know how he or she thinks or feels, and say something which hurts him or her.

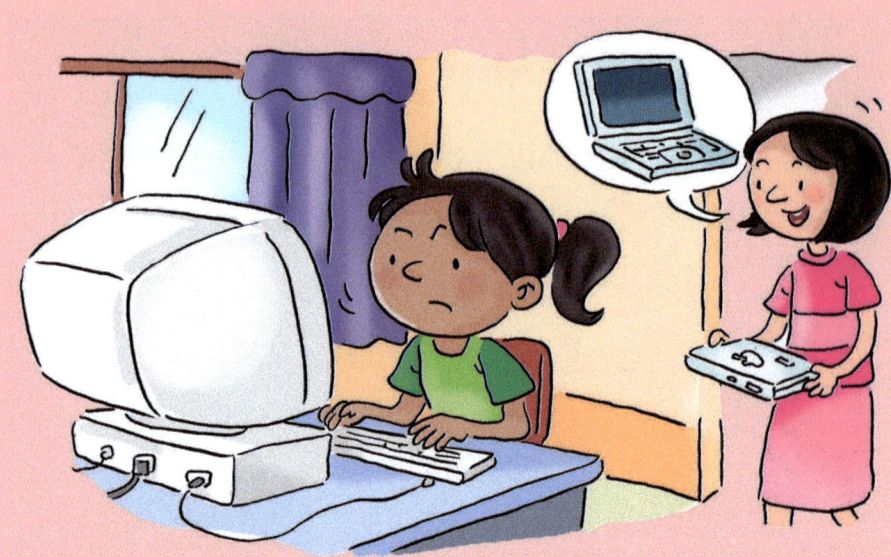

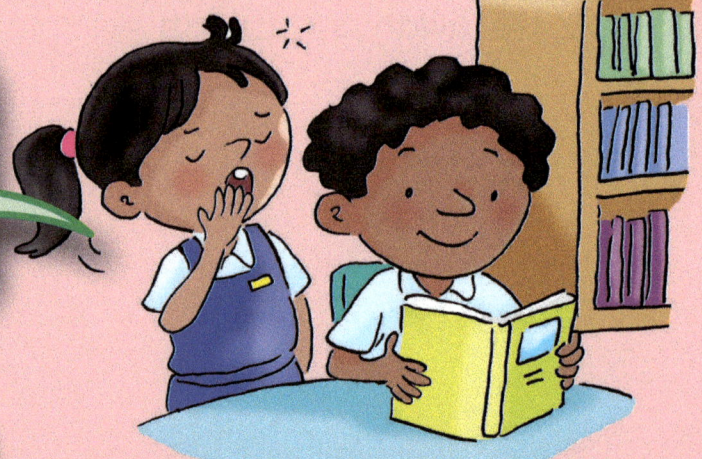

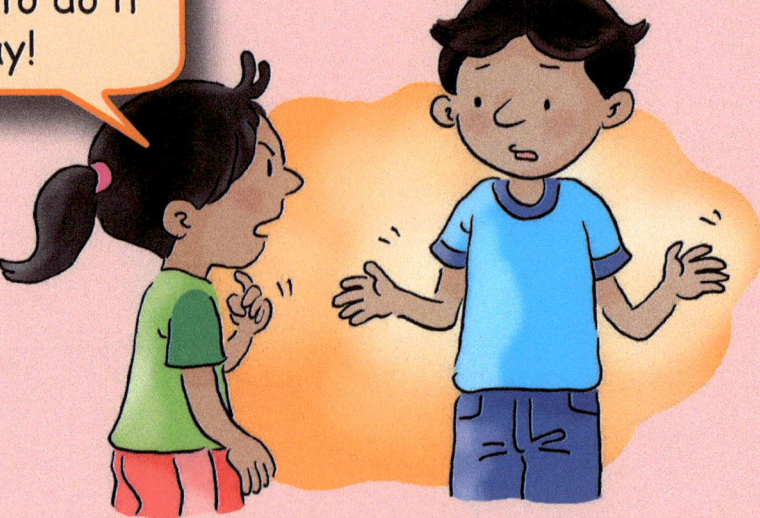

Name: Class: Date:

Lesson 3

What Started It?

There are many different causes for conflicts.

Below are some of the causes. Put a tick (✓) in the boxes if they had been the cause of conflict in the past for you.

1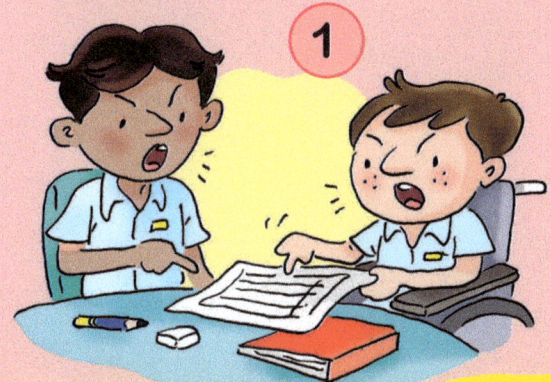
Arguing about who is right and wrong.

2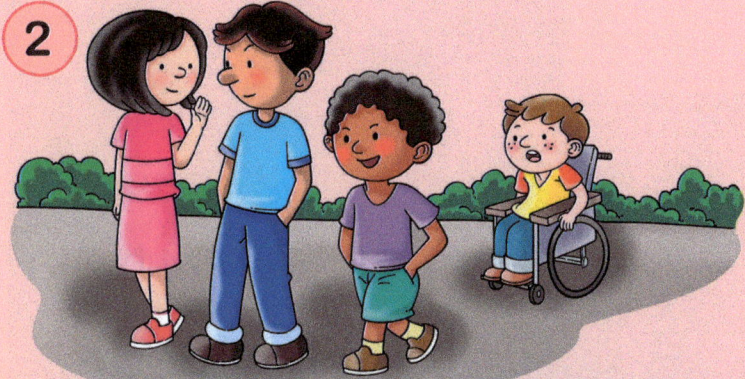
Getting others to leave someone out of the group.

3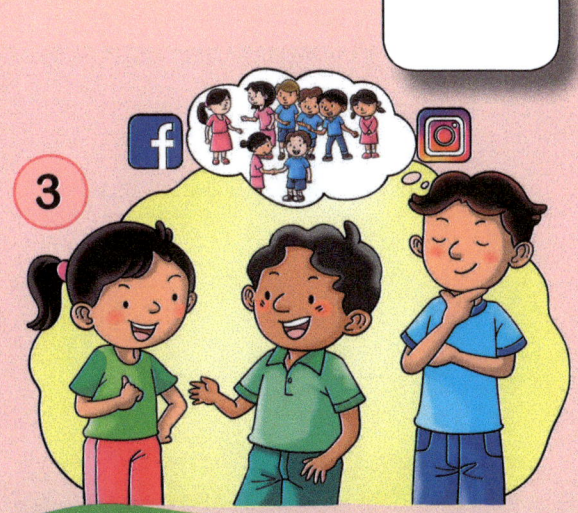
Comparing who has more friends.

4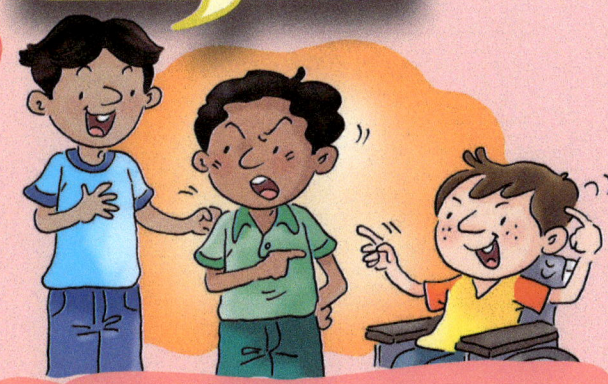
Do not take Harold seriously!
Calling names and insulting each other.

Learning Objective: Pupils will be able to understand how conflicts with others may be avoided or resolved.

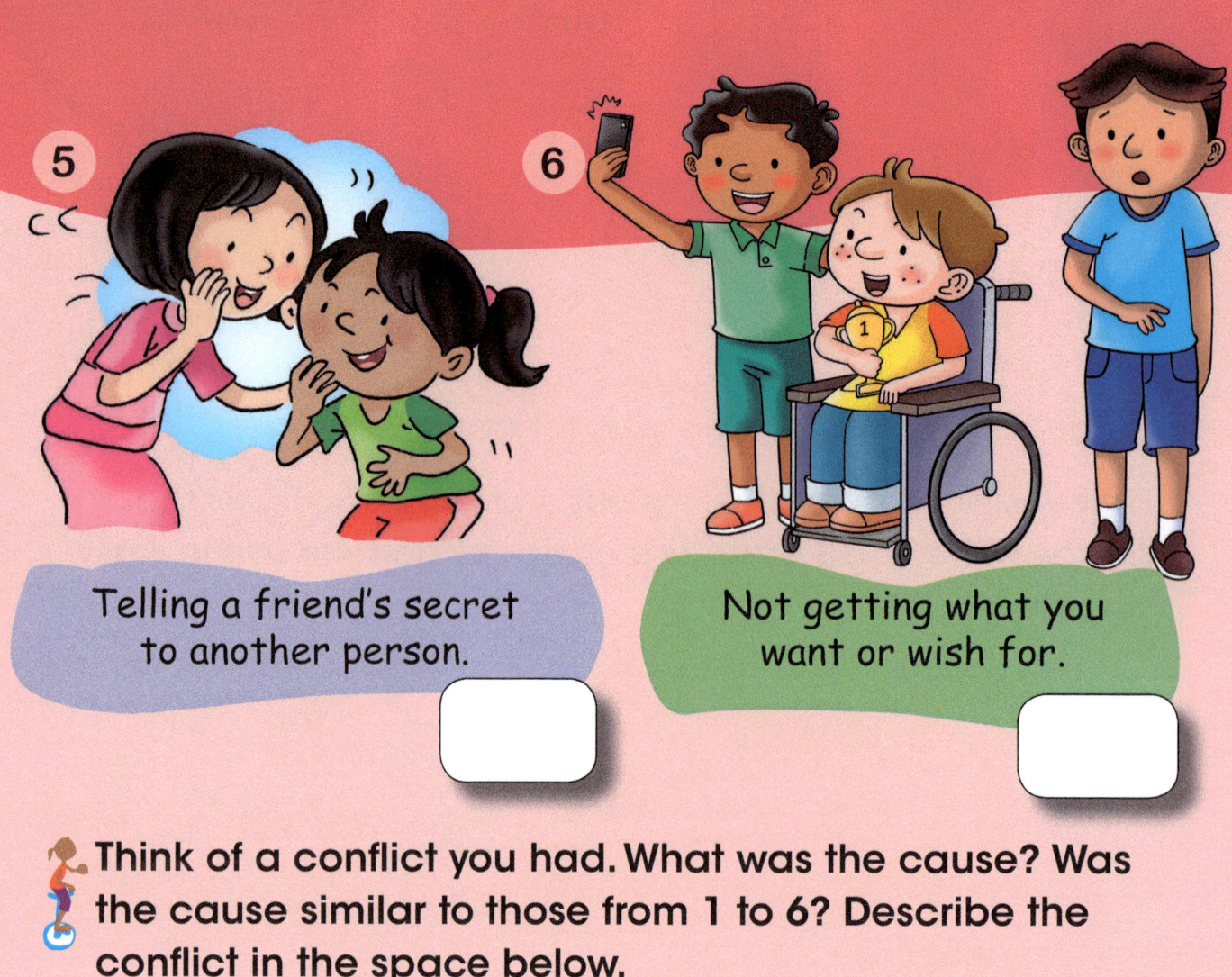

5 Telling a friend's secret to another person.

6 Not getting what you want or wish for.

Think of a conflict you had. What was the cause? Was the cause similar to those from 1 to 6? Describe the conflict in the space below.

Resolving Conflicts

Lesson 4

Name: Class: Date:

The superfriends are not happy with Ajit. Hidden in the maze are some things Ajit can say or do to help the friendship.

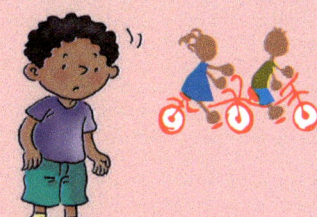

Circle the things Ajit can say or do. Then draw a line to connect him to the superfriends.

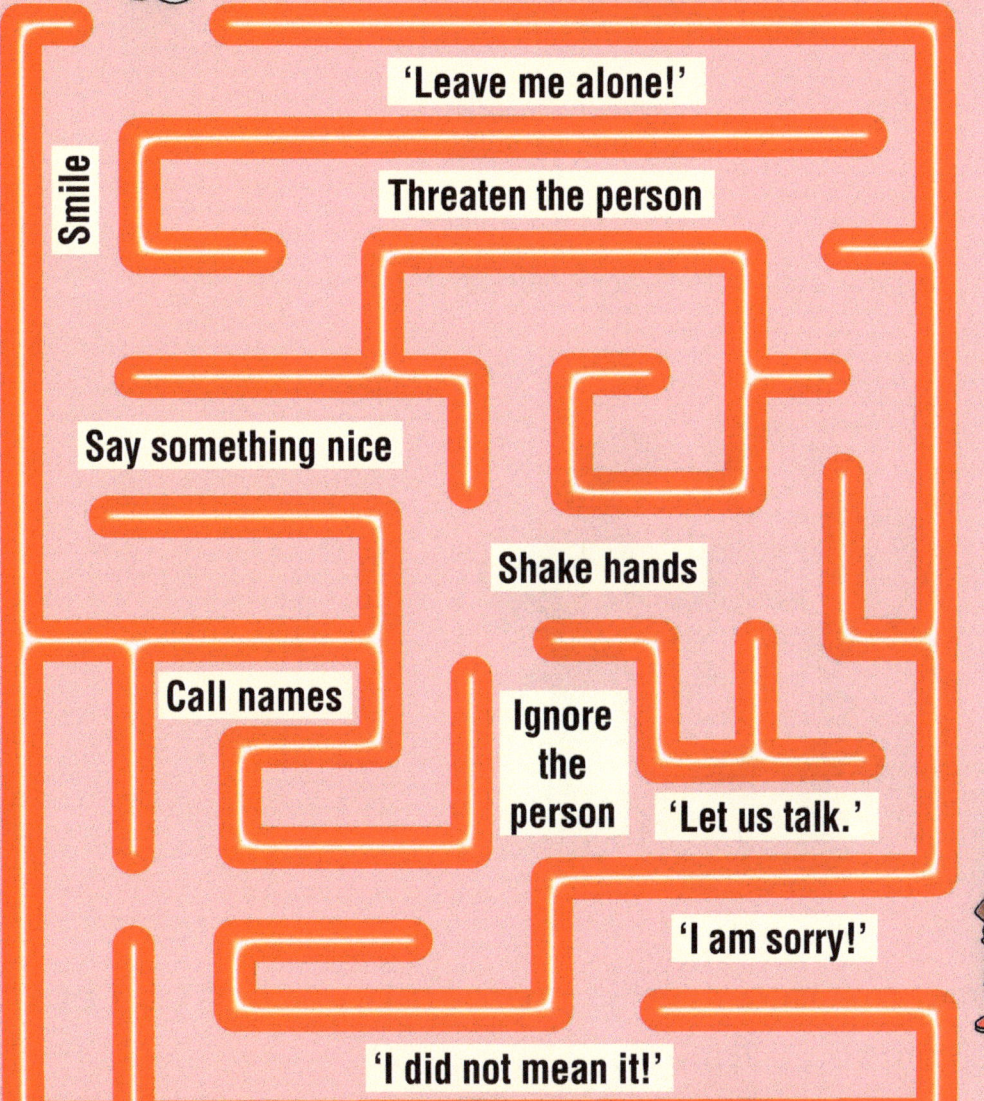

- Smile
- 'Leave me alone!'
- Threaten the person
- Say something nice
- Shake hands
- Call names
- Ignore the person
- 'Let us talk.'
- 'I am sorry!'
- 'I did not mean it!'

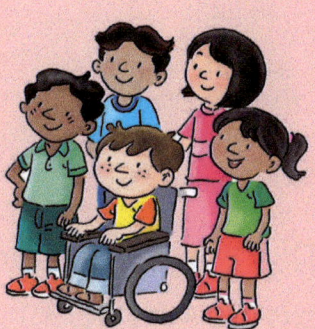

Learning Objective: Pupils will be able to understand how conflicts with others may be avoided or resolved.

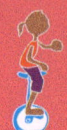 Which did you circle in the maze? Write them below.

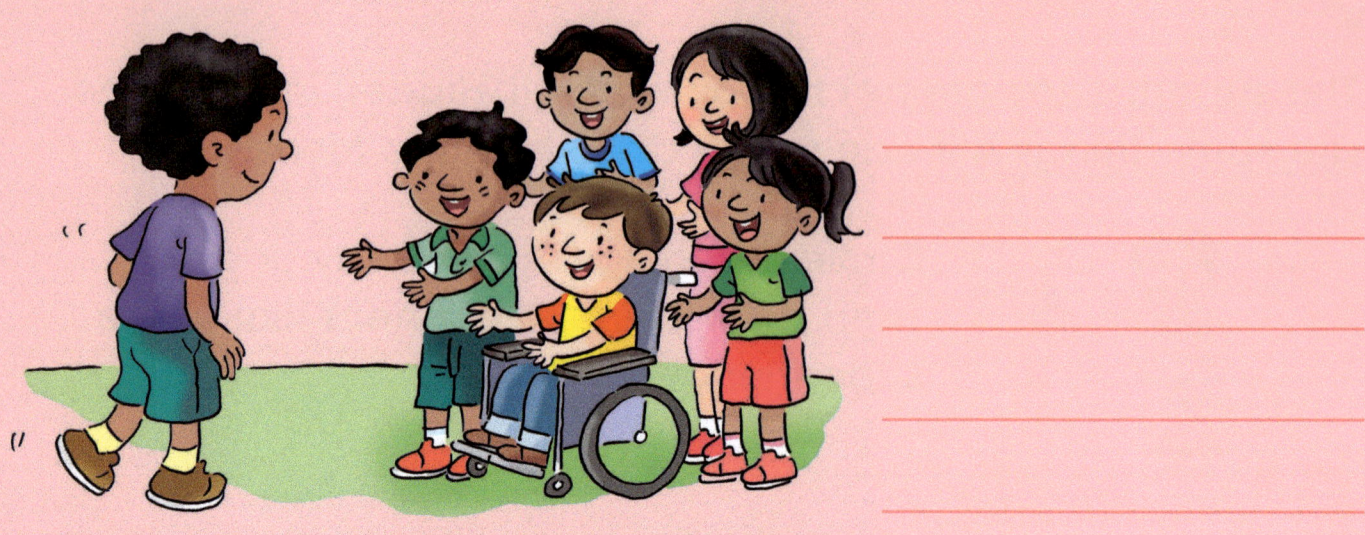

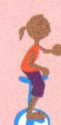 Which words were not circled? Write them below.

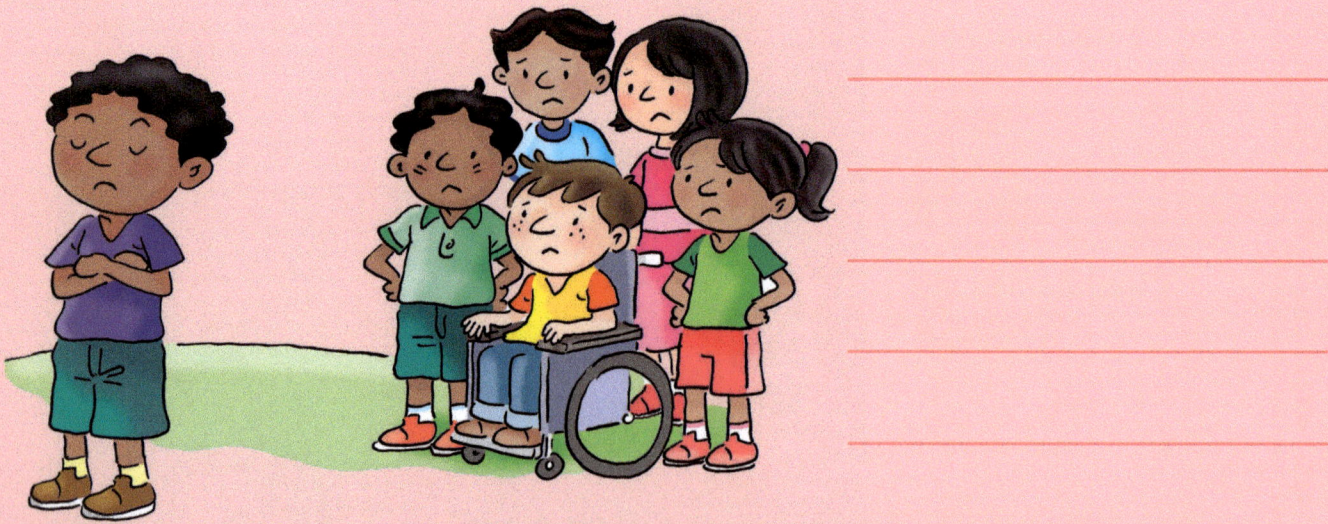

The next time you are in a conflict, remember what you can do or say to help resolve things.

resolve: to find a way of dealing with a problem or difficulty.

Name: 　　　　　　　　　Class: 　　　　Date: 　　　　　　　Lesson 5

No More Conflicts

When you are in conflict with someone, what do you do? Put a tick (✓) in the boxes.

1. I try to calm down before I speak.
2. I say how I feel. I do not care if it hurts the person.
3. I threaten the person I am arguing with.
4. I try to make peace with the person.
5. I smile and say something nice about the person.
6. I keep quiet, then agree with the person.
7. I hit the person so that I will feel better.
8. I say different things to different people so that they will support me.
9. I try and invite the person to join me in other activities.
10. I think about how the person feels.
11. I listen if the person wants to talk to me.
12. I shout at the person to make him scared of me.

Learning Objective: Pupils will be able to understand how conflicts with others may be avoided or resolved.

To resolve conflicts, we can start with the following:
Stop. Pause. Think. Do not respond immediately to words or actions we do not like.

These can help make your friends less angry too:
1. Smile.
2. Say 'I am sorry'.

Look at the pictures below. What should Harold and Lam say? Fill in the speech bubbles.

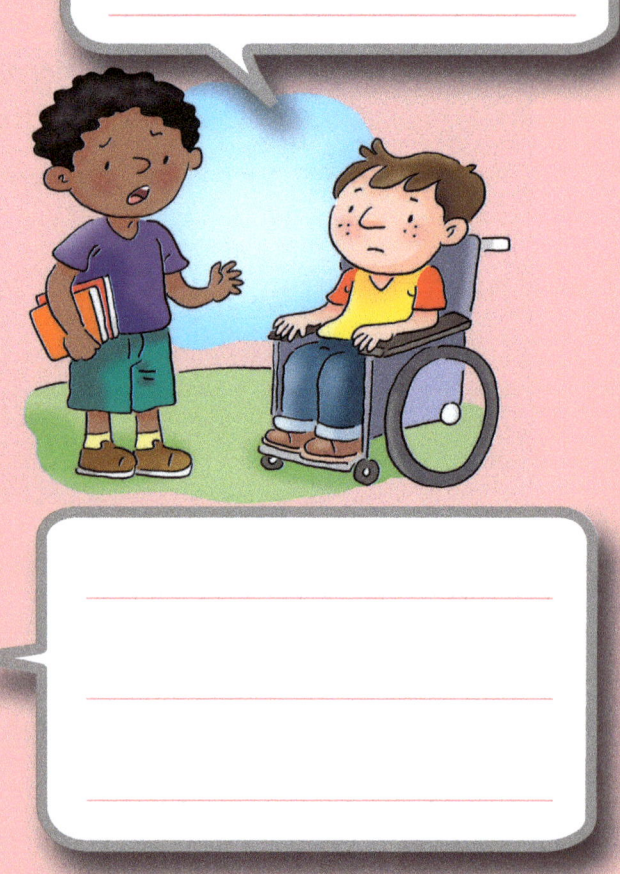

Why do you keep saying books are boring? Are you saying I am a boring person?

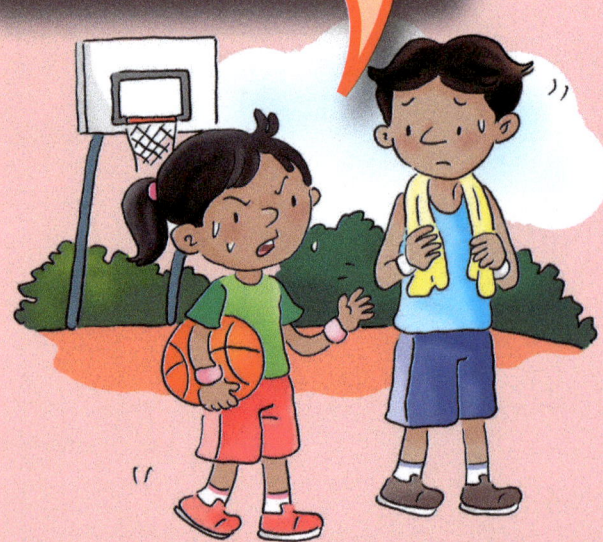

If you had passed the ball to Eileen, we could have won the game.

Practise and use these skills often. You may not get it right the first time but you will get better if you continue to work on them.

Name: Class: Date:

Lesson 6

I Do Not Feel Good

 Look at the pictures below. Tawan, Haris, Harold and Ajit do not feel good about themselves. Why do you think this is so?

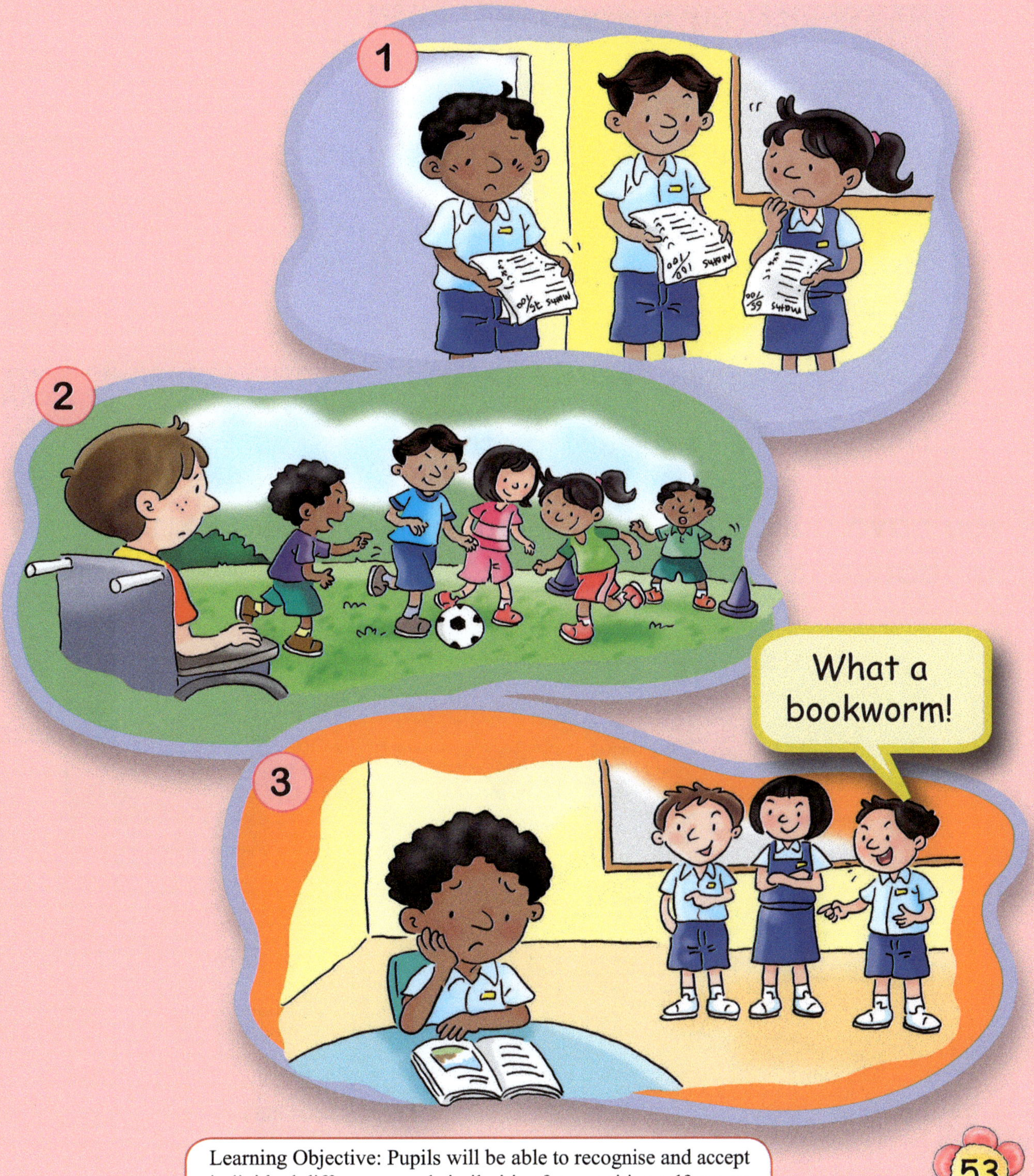

1

2

What a bookworm!

3

Learning Objective: Pupils will be able to recognise and accept individual differences and similarities for a positive self-esteem.

Read the statements below. Put a tick (✓) in the box if the statement describes you.

1. I often feel sad.
2. I find it difficult to feel happy.
3. I am often stressed and worried.
4. I feel lonely all the time.
5. I find it difficult to study or learn.
6. Everyone is smarter than me.
7. My parents love my brothers and sisters more than me.
8. I have very few friends because I do not look good.
9. I wish I have more friends in class.
10. I find it difficult to talk to others.

If you have put a tick (✓) in more than one box, speak to your teacher or counsellor.

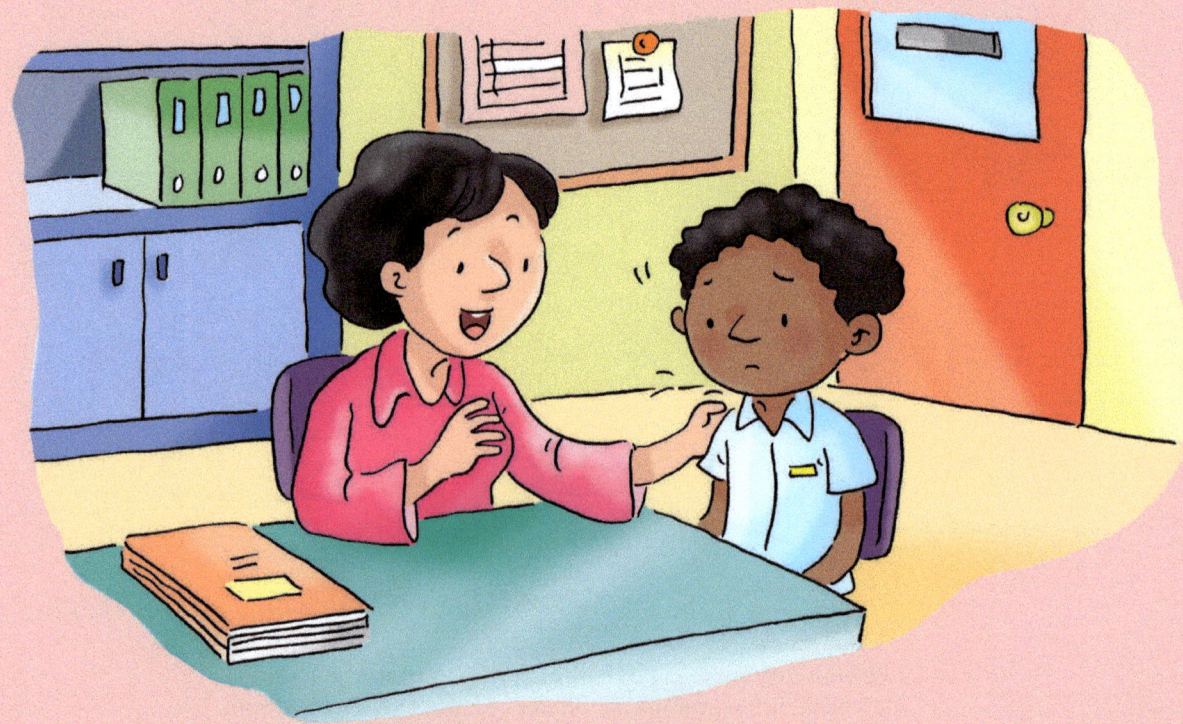

Name:　　　　　　　Class:　　　　　Date:

Lesson 7

Same Or Different?

The superfriends come from different countries. They are different in their own ways. However, the superfriends share have many things in common too. What are the things they have in common in pictures 1 to 6?

1

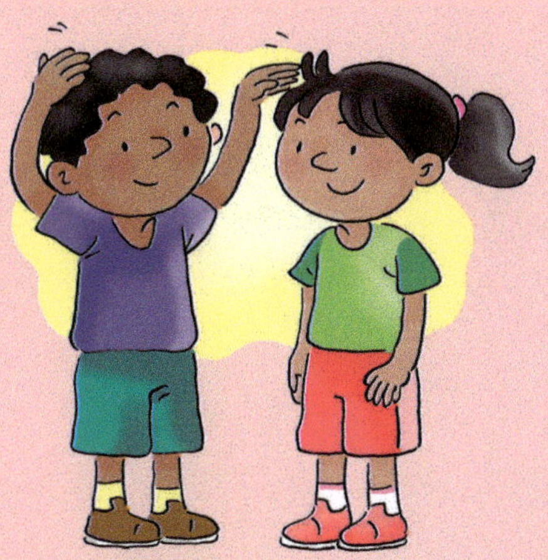

2

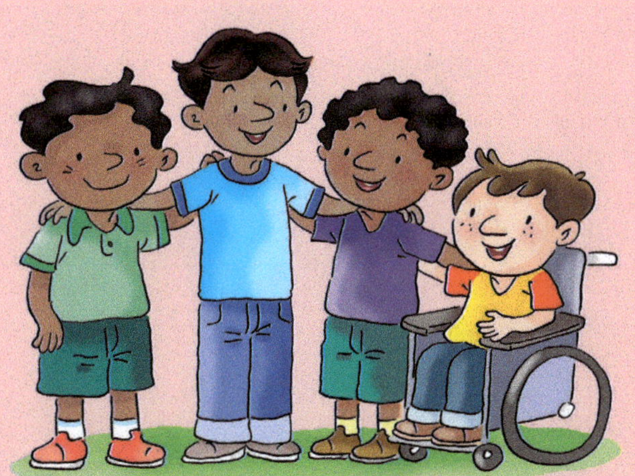

3

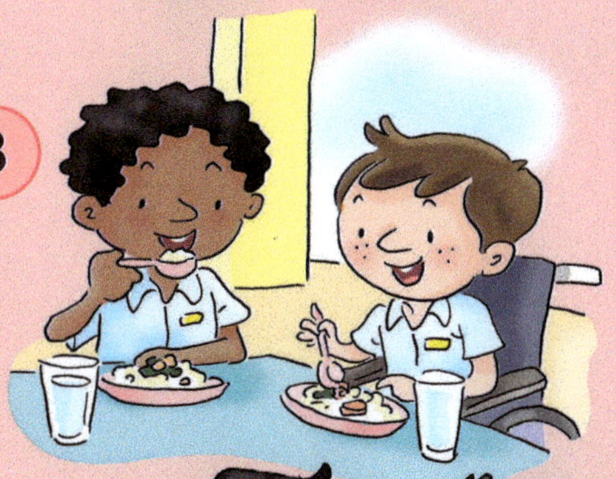

4

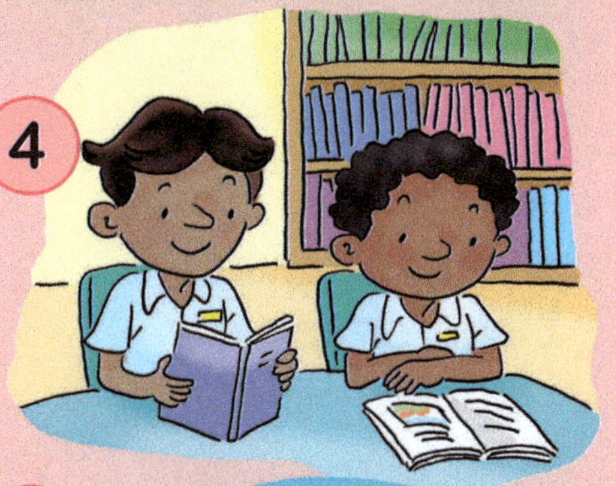

5

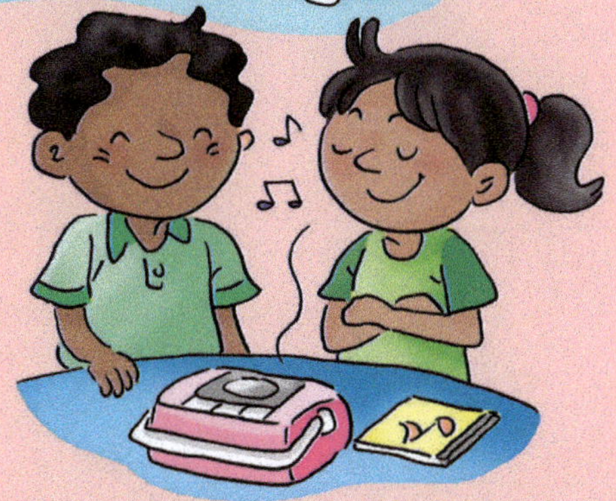

6

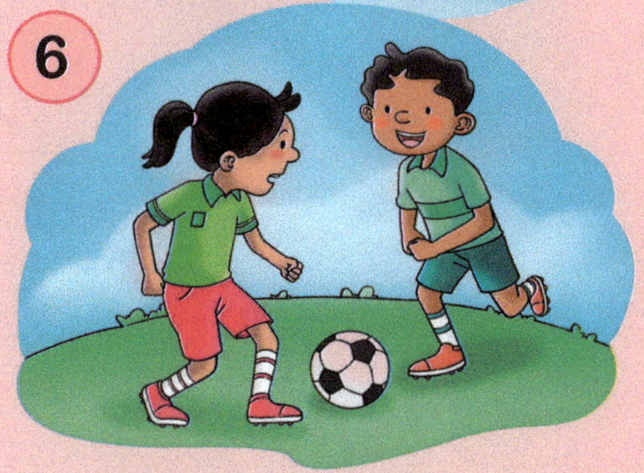

What do you have in common with your partner?
How are the both of you different?

Learning Objective: Pupils will be able to recognise and accept individual differences and similarities for a positive self-esteem.

55

It is perfectly fine to be different from your family and friends. Being different does not make them accept or love you less!

See how Eileen and Lam respond when they feel different from others.

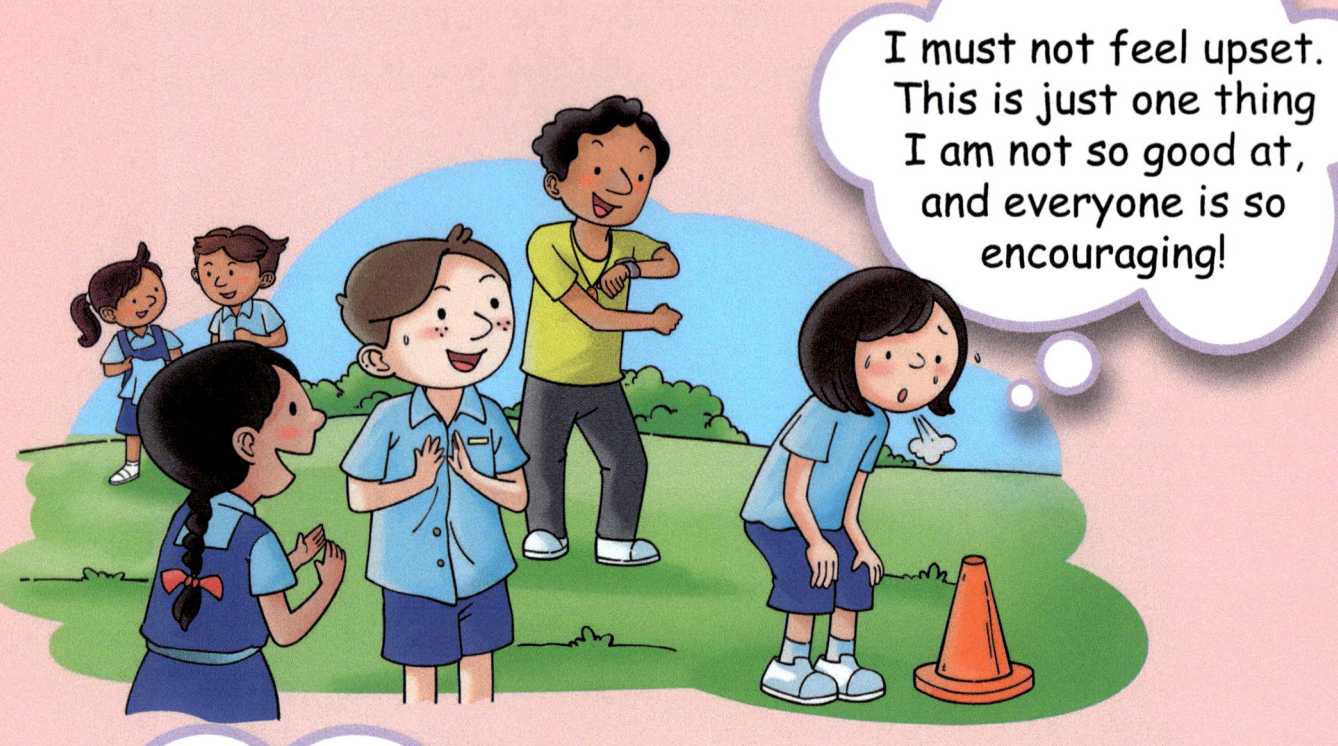

I must not feel upset. This is just one thing I am not so good at, and everyone is so encouraging!

I may not know how to swim, but I can cheer my friends on!

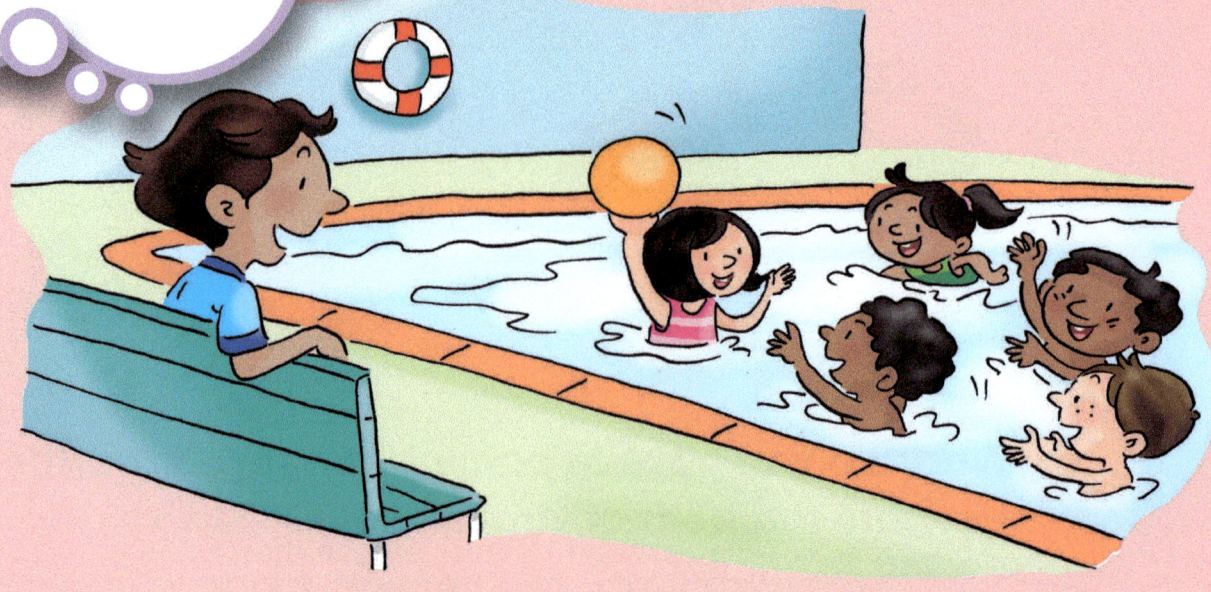

Name: Class: Date: Lesson 8

I Am Special

Read what makes Tawan, Harold, Lam and Ajit special.

1.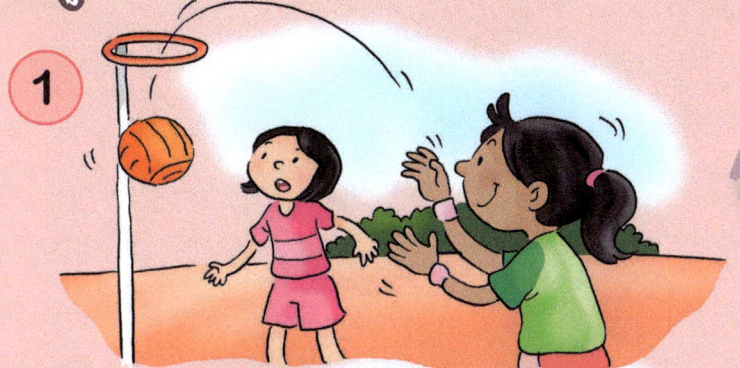

   I am good at sports and that makes me special!

2.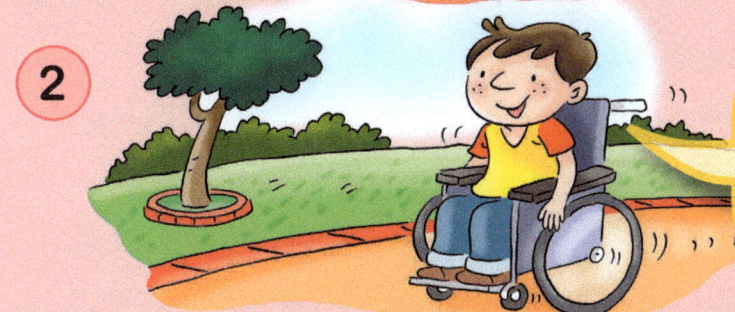

   I am special because I can get around on my own and make my friends happy!

3.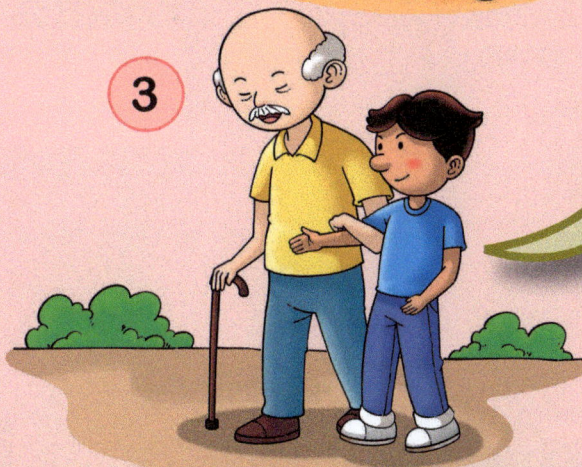

   Older people say I listen patiently when they talk to me. That makes me very special!

4.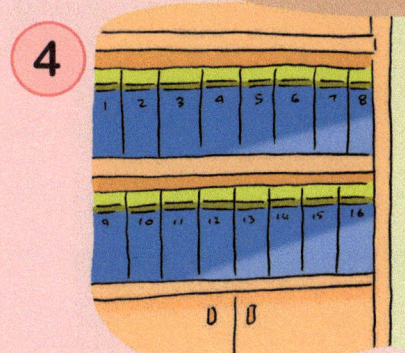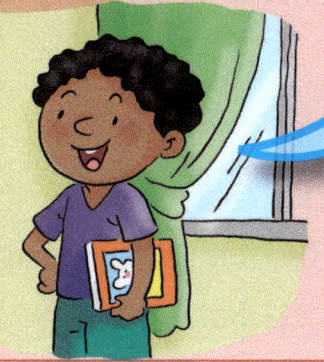

   I help my friends with their English and that makes me feel special!

Learning Objective: Pupils will be able to recognise and accept individual differences and similarities for a positive self-esteem.

All of us are special in our own ways. How are *you* special?

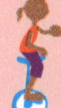
You may write or draw to show what makes you special. Here are the many adjectives you can use. You are also free to use other positive adjectives not found here.

polite   honest   strong   cheerful   kind   loyal
smart   encouraging   caring   brave   friendly   helpful
considerate   careful   humorous   peace-loving

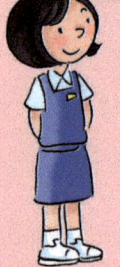
I am special because ...
_____
_____
_____
_____

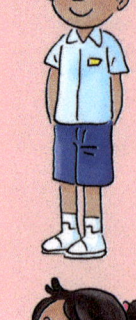

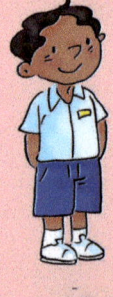

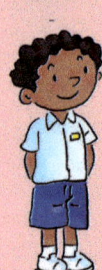

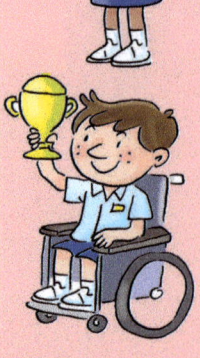

Actively listening to others makes the person talking to you feel special too. You have the power to make others feel good about themselves.

Name: Class: Date: Lesson 9

The Good, Bad And Ugly

Words and actions can show our care for others. Yet, sometimes what we say and do can also annoy others and make them feel bad.

Look at the pictures below. Circle the superfriends who are annoying and making others feel bad. Why do you think they are behaving badly?

1. "Hurry up and pass the ball to me!"

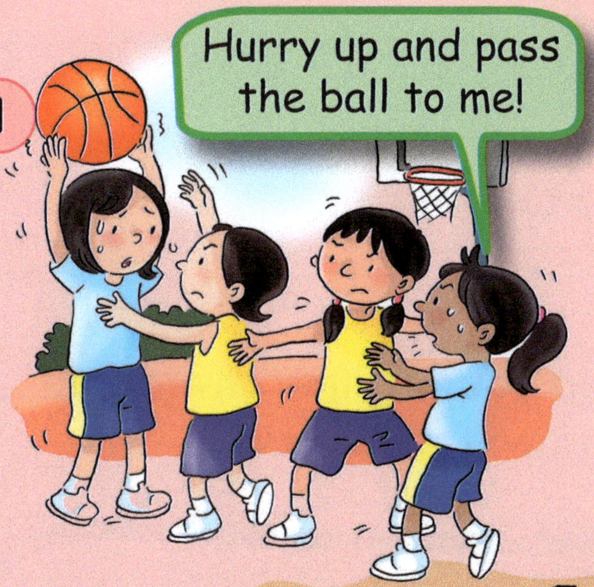

2.

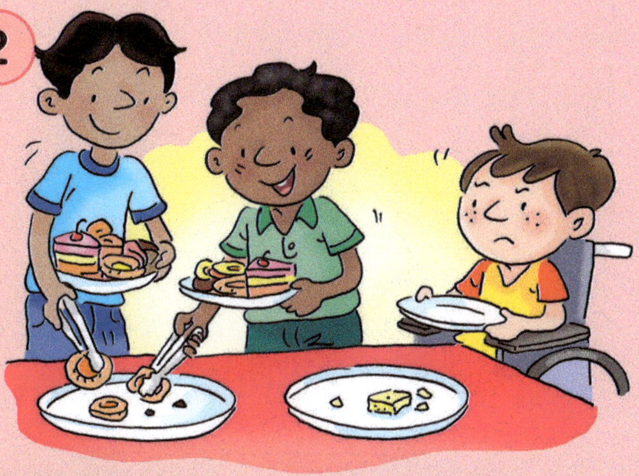

3. "Yippee! All these seats are ours!"

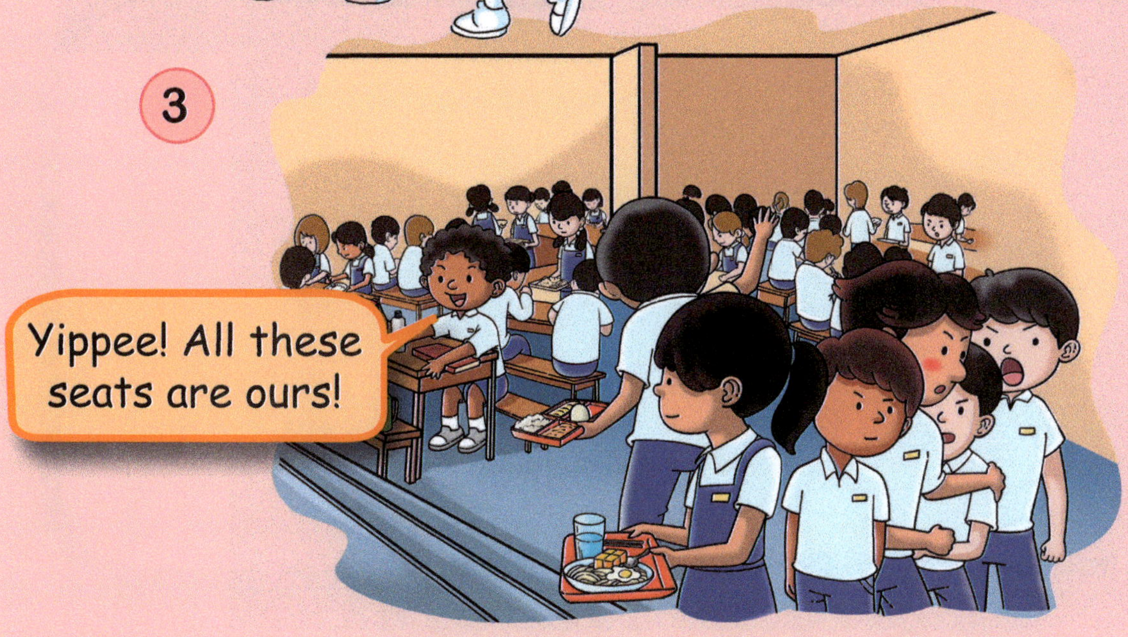

Learning Objective: Pupils will be able to recognise and accept individual differences and similarities for a positive self-esteem.

Sometimes we hurt others through our weaknesses. This is why we must try to overcome our own problems.

 Exchange your Pupil's Book with your partner. Think of one strength and one weakness your partner has and write them in his or her book.

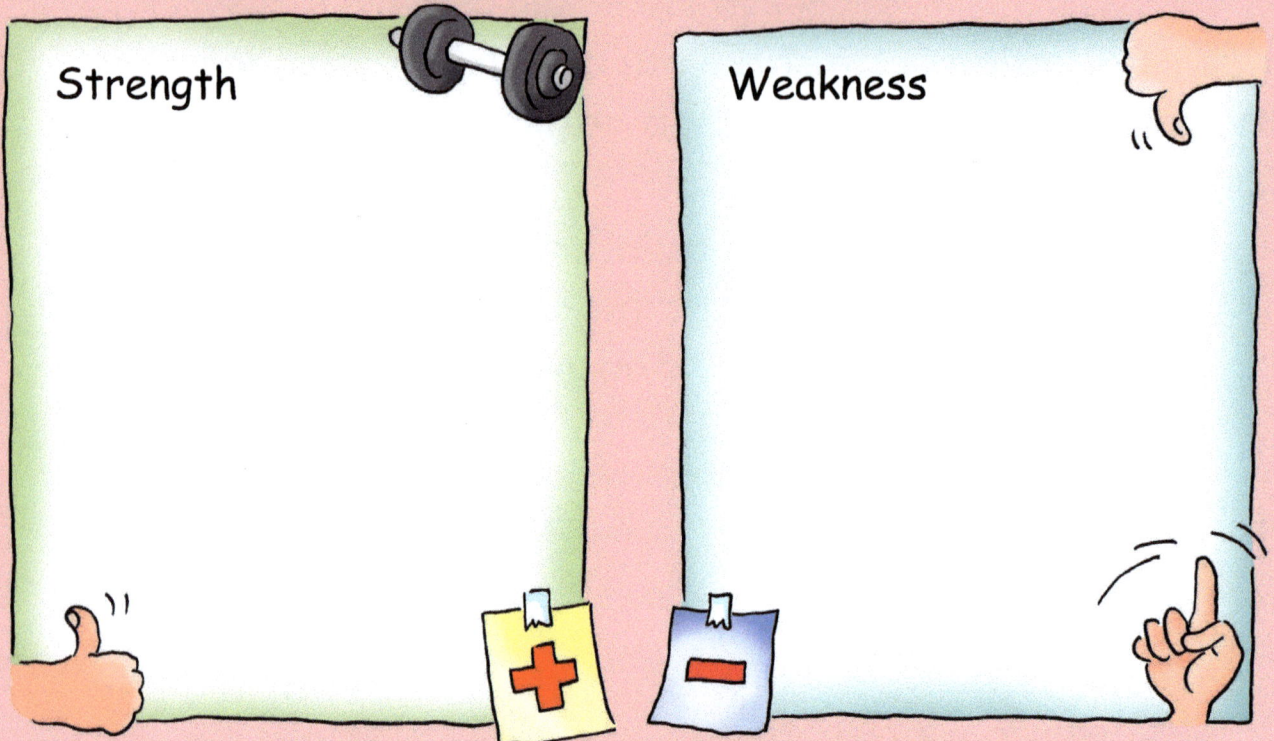

 Think of one way to help your partner overcome his or her weakness and write it below.

Try this!

overcome: to get rid of.

Name: Class: Date:

Lesson 10

My Special Shield

Remembering your strengths is one way to help you feel good about yourself.

Complete the sentences in the Special Shield below. Cut it out and keep it in your wallet. Read it the next time you do not feel good about yourself.

My friends say I am good at ...
_____
_____
_____

I am good at ...
_____
_____
_____

People tell me they like the way I ...
_____
_____
_____

I try very hard at ...
_____
_____
_____

Learning Objective: Pupils will be able to recognise and accept individual differences and similarities for a positive self-esteem.

This page is left blank for the cutting exercise on the previous page.

Name: Class: Date: Lesson 11

Building Relationships

Having good relationships with people can help you feel good about yourself.

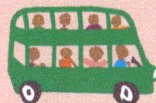 Look at the pictures below. Discuss what Tawan, Haris, Lam and Eileen are doing.

1

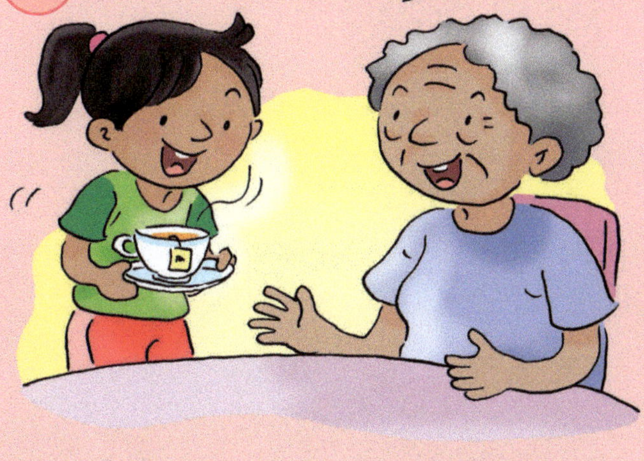

2

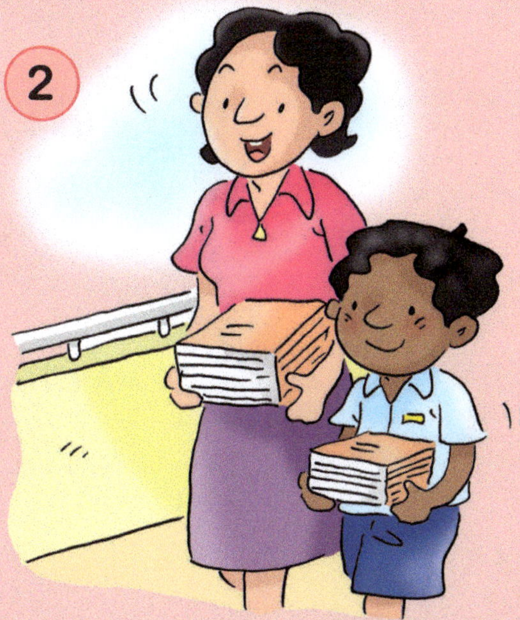

3

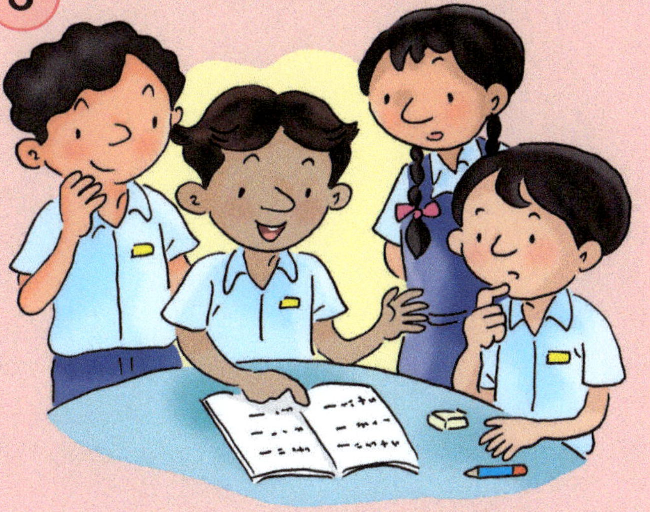

4

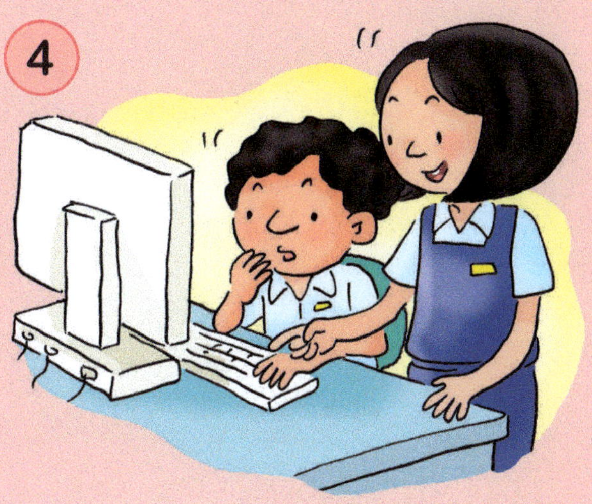

Learning Objective: Pupils will be able to recognise that establishing good relationships can build positive self-esteem.

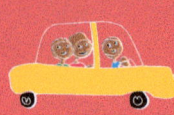 Think of four ways you can build a good relationship with your friends and family members. List them below.

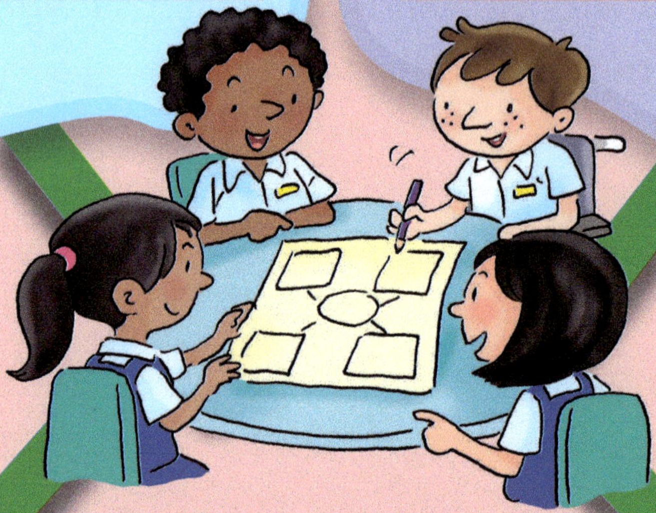

Relationship keepers and builders

MY LEARNING LOG

NEW WORDS

Lesson: ___ Date: ___
MY LESSON TODAY …
(Draw or write out the things you remember.)

Lesson: ___ Date: ___
MY LESSON TODAY …
(Draw or write out the things you remember.)

Lesson: ___ Date: ___
MY LESSON TODAY …
(Draw or write out the things you remember.)

Lesson: ___ Date: ___
MY LESSON TODAY …
(Draw or write out the things you remember.)

Lesson: ___ Date: ___
MY LESSON TODAY …
(Draw or write out the things you remember.)

MY LEARNING LOG

NEW WORDS

Lesson: Date:

MY LESSON TODAY …
(Draw or write out the things you remember.)

Lesson: Date:

MY LESSON TODAY …
(Draw or write out the things you remember.)

Lesson: Date:

MY LESSON TODAY …
(Draw or write out the things you remember.)

Lesson: Date:

MY LESSON TODAY …
(Draw or write out the things you remember.)

Lesson: Date:

MY LESSON TODAY …
(Draw or write out the things you remember.)

MY LEARNING LOG

NEW WORDS

Lesson: ___ Date: ___

MY LESSON TODAY …
(Draw or write out the things you remember.)

Lesson: ___ Date: ___

MY LESSON TODAY …
(Draw or write out the things you remember.)

Lesson: ___ Date: ___

MY LESSON TODAY …
(Draw or write out the things you remember.)

Lesson: ___ Date: ___

MY LESSON TODAY …
(Draw or write out the things you remember.)

Lesson: ___ Date: ___

MY LESSON TODAY …
(Draw or write out the things you remember.)

MY LEARNING LOG

NEW WORDS

Lesson: Date:

MY LESSON TODAY …
(Draw or write out the things you remember.)

Lesson: Date:

MY LESSON TODAY …
(Draw or write out the things you remember.)

Lesson: Date:

MY LESSON TODAY …
(Draw or write out the things you remember.)

Lesson: Date:

MY LESSON TODAY …
(Draw or write out the things you remember.)

Lesson: Date:

MY LESSON TODAY …
(Draw or write out the things you remember.)

NEW WORDS

Lesson: **Date:**

MY LESSON TODAY ...
(Draw or write out the things you remember.)

Lesson: **Date:**

MY LESSON TODAY ...
(Draw or write out the things you remember.)

Lesson: **Date:**

MY LESSON TODAY ...
(Draw or write out the things you remember.)

Lesson: **Date:**

MY LESSON TODAY ...
(Draw or write out the things you remember.)

Lesson: **Date:**

MY LESSON TODAY ...
(Draw or write out the things you remember.)

MY LEARNING LOG

MY LEARNING LOG

NEW WORDS

Lesson: ____ Date: ____

MY LESSON TODAY …
(Draw or write out the things you remember.)

Lesson: ____ Date: ____

MY LESSON TODAY …
(Draw or write out the things you remember.)

Lesson: ____ Date: ____

MY LESSON TODAY …
(Draw or write out the things you remember.)

Lesson: ____ Date: ____

MY LESSON TODAY …
(Draw or write out the things you remember.)

Lesson: ____ Date: ____

MY LESSON TODAY …
(Draw or write out the things you remember.)

Hachette UK's policy is to use papers that are natural, renewable and recyclable products and made from wood grown in well-managed forests and other controlled sources. The logging and manufacturing processes are expected to conform to the environmental regulations of the country of origin.

ISBN: 978 981 47 6774 3

© Dr Michael Chia 2007, 2018

First published in 2007 by Pearson Education South Asia Pte Ltd

This new edition published in 2018 by
Hachette Singapore Private Limited
Published from 2023 by Hodder Education,
An Hachette UK Company
Carmelite House
50 Victoria Embankment
London EC4Y 0DZ
www.hoddereducation.com

Impression number   10 9 8 7 6 5
Year   2023

All rights reserved. Apart from any use permitted under UK copyright law, no part of this publication may be reproduced or transmitted in any form or by any means, electronic or mechanical, including photocopying and recording, or held within any information storage and retrieval system, without permission in writing from the publisher or under licence from the Copyright Licensing Agency Limited. Further details of such licences (for reprographic reproduction) may be obtained from the Copyright Licensing Agency Limited, www.cla.co.uk

Printed by CPI Group (UK) Ltd, Croydon CR0 4YY

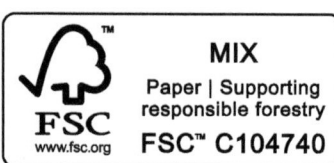